Food in Focus

Ann Carter *BA DipHealthEd CertEd*

Ann Carter has a wide experience in health education, and in teaching adults and young people in the UK and overseas. She worked in Stockport Health Promotion Unit as Programme Co-ordinator for the Stockport Community Smoking Prevention Programme from 1984 to 1987. Prior to this appointment, Ann worked on a special project aimed at preventing heart disease in the Newport area of Inner Middlesborough. She trains tutors for the Health Education Authority's 'Look After Yourself!' courses and has recently started a training and health promotion consultancy.

Sheila Bell *SRD*

Sheila Bell is a state registered dietitian, a member of the British Dietetic Association and its associated community nutrition group. She is also a tutor for the Health Education Authority's 'Look After Yourself!' courses. For a number of years, Sheila has worked in hospitals as a dietitian. As the project dietitian on a community health programme, she was involved in developing healthy eating initiatives with groups ranging from school children to the elderly.

Food in Focus
A Nutrition Education Programme for Health Educators

Ann Carter BA DipHealthEd CertEd

Sheila Bell SRD

An H M + M Publication

JOHN WILEY & SONS
Chichester · New York · Brisbane · Toronto · Singapore

H M + M Publishers is an imprint of John Wiley & Sons Ltd, Baffins Lane, Chichester, Sussex
PO19 1UD, England.

British Library Cataloguing in Publication Data

Carter, Ann
  Food in focus: a nutrition education
  programme for health educators.
  1. Nutrition — Study and teaching
  I. Title II. Bell, Sheila
  613.2'07   TX364

  ISBN 0 471 91746 X

Library of Congress Cataloging-in-Publication Data

Carter, Ann
  Food in focus.

  An H M + M publication.
  Bibliography: p.
  1. Nutrition—Study and teaching. I. Bell, Sheila.
II. Title. [DNLM: 1. Allied Health Personnel—
education. 2. Nutrition—education. 3. Teaching.
QU 18 C323f]
TX364.C375 1988   613.2'07'1   87 – 21553

  ISBN 0 471 91746 X (pbk.)

Typeset by Woodfield Graphics, Fontwell, Arundel, West Sussex.
Printed and bound in Great Britain by Anchor Brendon, Tiptree, Essex

Contents

Preface vii

Acknowledgements ix

Introduction 1

Session One 11
    Session plan 14
    How to play the Healthy Eating card game 17
    Name that Food! 29
    Food and drink diary 31

Session Two 33
    Session plan 36
    Is it your choice? 39
    Appraising your food and drink diary 40
    Finding your way round a label 44

Session Three 47
    Session plan 50
    Why less sugar? 53
    'A day in the life . . .' 54
    Going shopping 57
    The salt picture 58

Session Four 63
    Session plan 66
    Dietary fibre 68
    'Mix and match' 70
    Dietary fibre in your food 72

Session Five 75
   Session plan.. 78
   Fat—where are you? 80
   Fat—who needs it?.. 81
   'Fatty dip'.. 82
   Making and tasting healthy dishes 85

Session Six 87
   Session plan.. 90
   Food presentation.. 95

Session Seven 97
   Session plan.. 100

Bibliography 103

Preface

In September 1983, the National Advisory Committee for Nutrition Education (NACNE) published its proposals for nutritional guidelines for health education in Britain and these were closely followed by the publication of the report *Diet and Cardiovascular Disease* from the Committee on Medical Aspects of Food Policy (COMA) in 1984. Both these reports have laid down guidelines which recommend healthier ways of eating by the British public for the remainder of this century.

Since the publication of these two reports, there has been an upsurge of interest in healthy eating. The media coverage has been very comprehensive and may well have played a large part in the promotion of the current interest in food and health. New books have been published which have focused on 'eating for health'; and more cookery books have been coming on to the market which also emphasise the health aspects of food preparation and cooking.

In the face of all this publicity, the authors realised there was still a gap to be filled in the availability of educational materials to cater for the needs of professionals and public who wanted to put the new guidelines into practice in their daily lives. It was in order to meet this need that *Food in Focus* was written. It is a basic nutrition education resource designed for use by professionals who are running nutrition education programmes for their colleagues, members of the public, and young people in schools, and is centred on the current nutritional guidelines. It is not intended to provide yet another book about healthy eating; such books already provide useful resources and background information for running *Food in Focus* programmes.

The authors wish every success to those using *Food in Focus*. They hope that leaders and group members will enjoy using the materials as much as they have.

ANN CARTER
SHEILA BELL

Acknowledgements

The authors would like to thank the following: South Tees Health Authority for the support given by the Health Education Department and the Department of Nutrition and Dietetics; Stockport Health Authority for the interest and encouragement of the Health Promotion Unit; colleagues who have been involved in piloting courses and testing materials; all our friends and colleagues, without whose interest and encouragement *Food in Focus* would not have been completed; and Miss Jane Randall and Dr John Brown of the former Health Education Council for their advice and helpful criticism in preparing the final script.

The publishers are indebted to Churchill Livingstone for permission to reprint the height/weight chart from Garrow J (1981) *Treat Obesity Seriously* used in Session Six, and to Michael Kindred and Malcolm Goldsmith for the use of the 'Tour of Knowledge' Card Game idea devised by them (Patent No. 1601216) and used in the Healthy Eating Card Game in Session One.

INTRODUCTION

Introduction

The *Food in Focus* nutrition education programme consists of seven sessions, each of one-and-a-half hours' duration.

The Aims of the Programme

1   To develop the concept of healthy eating.
2   To create an awareness of some possible benefits of healthy eating, not only in promoting 'good health' but in preventing problems associated with certain diseases.
3   To create an awareness of the food-labelling system which currently operates in Britain and its implications for healthy eating.
4   To develop an understanding of the current nutritional recommendations relating to fat, fibre, salt and sugar.
5   To enable individuals to make appropriate changes to their personal eating patterns.

The Approach

Participatory learning methods are used throughout the programme. This particular way of working means that the emphasis is placed on learning through the continual involvement of group members in structured activities. Thus, the knowledge and experience of both group members and leader are fully utilised. An overview of the methods used in the course is given later in this Introduction in the section 'Participatory Learning in Groups'.

The Content

The programme content promotes healthy eating: it does not deal in any way with slimming, crash diets or methods which promote rapid weight loss. The material helps group members to monitor, assess and change their eating patterns within individual life styles. In order to do this, the material encourages the interpretation of food labels and the application of the current nutritional recommendations to fat, fibre, salt and sugar. The health implications of the recommendations are considered in some detail. Group members are encouraged to relate the content of each session to making healthy food choices in their daily lives. Perceptions of a healthy weight are discussed towards the end of the course. The final session brings together the knowledge and skills acquired on the course through an integrated group project.

The course material is designed to be flexible and can easily be adapted to meet group needs. Although each session is planned to last for one-and-a-half hours, variations in the time available can easily be catered for by varying the content and detail presented in each session.

Using the Programme

Each section of the programme contains a guide, a session plan, group material and leader's material. Details of each of these components is listed below.

(a) *The Guide*

This states the contents, the aids required and the objectives for each session, and presents a brief overview of the activities.

(b) *Session Plan*

The plan gives the timetable for the session. It outlines the activities and their approximate timing.

(c) *Group Material*

This is for use by group members and is usually in the form of task sheets. It may be photocopied, where appropriate, so that it is readily available for use.

(d) *Leader's Material*

This is intended as background information for the group leader. It outlines the main learning points for each session, and provides instructions on how to carry out the activities and information to help with their debriefing. The latter is usually presented in the form of a 'checklist'.

The materials recommended for use in each session are provided in the manual. Group leaders may wish to supplement this material where it is appropriate to the needs of the group.

Target Groups

The programme has been extensively piloted with a variety of target groups. It has been designed for use primarily with adults, and is also suitable for use as resource material for young people aged thirteen and upwards. Although the approach is suitable for any group, the content needs to be varied to meet the requirements of very specific target groups, eg. the elderly, people with special dietary problems, and those needing information about infant nutrition. The programme can be used with people from a variety of cultures or ethnic backgrounds.

Developing the Programme

Professionals using *Food in Focus* will probably identify certain areas of the programme which could be developed for use with a variety of target groups.

The course could be used as a foundation for groups who, for example, meet in connection with the implementation of food policies in industry. It could be used for inclusion in women's health courses and by those involved in running weight-loss and weight-gain groups. The material is also useful as a resource by tutors who are involved in running the Health Education Authority's 'Look After Yourself!' course. School teachers will find the material especially versatile. The contents may be used as a complete course, or particular sessions or activities may be incorporated into an existing syllabus. Once professionals have familiarised themselves with the approach and the content, they will be able to see for themselves how the material could be developed and used to its best advantage.

Participatory Learning in Groups

Participatory learning enables the leader and group members to become involved in the learning process through a mutual sharing of information and experience. Throughout the session, open communication is maintained between the leader and the group; the members are encouraged to interact and learn from one another. This approach to learning is rather different from some more traditional teaching methods which may be of a didactic nature. However, as one becomes more familiar with participatory learning, the process can be very enjoyable for all concerned.

When running *Food in Focus* programmes the authors find it useful to commence the sessions with themselves and the group members sitting in a circle. The formation of a circle encourages eye contact and interpersonal communication. Everyone is afforded the same status in the group, including the leader who is also part of the circle. As the group embarks on its various activities, the circle will be broken, but will need to re-form for the feedback from the exercises and for full group discussions.

The following notes provide details of the methods used in *Food in Focus*. As one becomes more experienced in this way of working, it is likely that other activities will be devised to meet the needs of specific groups.

Ground Rules

Ground rules are the foundations on which the group operates its sessions. Some ground rules may be stated by the leader at the commencement of a programme of work, others may be negotiated as the group progresses, and some may be hidden and never openly stated.

When starting the first session of a course, leaders may like to consider making some of the following as ground rules for their sessions:

(a)   The sessions will start promptly and finish at a stated time.
(b)   Group members are to contribute at a level with which they are comfortable. They need only share as much as they wish to disclose.

(c)   One person at a time is to speak in discussions.
(d)   Everyone's contribution is to be equally valued.

The above suggestions are some which the authors have found useful in running groups. Ground rules are an essential part of group life and it is often useful to remind the group members of them at an appropriate time by asking "What are the ground rules which are operating in this group?".

Warm-up Activities

Such activities are generally used at the beginning of a session. They have one or more of the following functions:

(a)   to enable group members to get to know each other at the start of the course;
(b)   to bring individuals together as a group after a period of time apart;
(c)   to act as a 'leveller'—especially where group members are from a variety of professional or cultural backgrounds;
(d)   to provide an introduction to the work of the session.

In *Food in Focus*, the warm-up activities are based on the full circle. In Session One, the group members are asked to introduce themselves to the group. This is a quick and easy ice-breaker which is followed by an activity which will reinforce the interaction process and getting to know who is who. The 'Name Game' in Session Two is also a warm-up, and an example of how the exercise is carried out is given below.

The Name Game

The person in the group who is to start says "My name is Jack". The person to the right (or left) of Jack says "My name is Ann and this is Jack". The person next to Ann then says "My name is Mandy, this is Ann and this is Jack". This process operates until everyone has had his turn. The group members who go last may feel a little anxious. If the group is large, sixteen names is quite a task to repeat. Leaders need to reassure the group that the members can act as prompts and it is often useful if leaders are prepared to put themselves 'on trial' and say the last round of names themselves.

In future sessions in the programme, warm-ups are part of the session's work. Other activities of this nature may be introduced at the discretion of the leader, depending on the time available.

Warm-up activities are useful but not essential. When used they need to be kept brief and to the point. Ten minutes is possibly long enough to spend on a warm-up activity unless it is designed to be an integral part of the session.

Other ideas for warm-up activities may be found in *The Gamester's Handbook* (see Bibliography).

Brainstorming

The purpose of this activity is to generate many ideas on a topic in a short period of time. These ideas may be used to promote discussion and/or act as a starting point for future activities.

Group members are asked to call out whatever ideas about a particular topic come into their heads. The leader writes the ideas on a flip-chart/overhead projector (OHP). There are no comments at this stage—remarks anyone wishes to make should be left until the exercise is discussed.

It is better to look for a quantitiy of ideas rather than quality. Initially, there is no place for a 'wrong answer'. If the brainstorm is properly led, everyone has a chance to contribute and feels that his idea is worth writing down. As all ideas are valid, it channels the group away from a competitive atmosphere in which individuals compete to have their own ideas accepted. The activity becomes a collaborative one rather than one where a few group members dominate the activity.

Brainstorming can be a useful exercise, but group leaders need to be aware of the need for regulating the speed at which the ideas are presented. It is impossible to write down more than one idea at a time!

Rounds

A round is a process by which each person in turn, progressing round the full group circle, makes a statement which is relevant to an activity or situation.

Anyone can start a round. It does not have to be the leader or the person next to the leader. The person who starts usually decides whether the round will go clockwise or anticlockwise. Statements should be kept brief; it can be very boring to be at the end of a round which has taken an hour to complete.

Rounds very often start with an open-ended statement. For example, in Session One the group is asked to complete a round of ''One thing I learned from playing the card game is . . .''. Other openers for rounds are ''I discovered . . .'', ''I wish . . .'', ''I learned . . .'', ''I noticed . . .'', ''I regret . . .''. Rounds may be used to find out what the group noticed from watching a film, in evaluating a course or an activity, to express opinions, to give feedback or to start discussions. The use of rounds is endless and they provide a very useful activity to allow for the expression of the range of opinions, ideas and feelings which exist in a group.

It is important to emphasise the 'rules' of this activity. Group members listen to the statement which is being made. Comments should not be made until the round is over. If a statement does warrant discussion, it should be saved until the end of the round. It is very easy for a round to become a general discussion if group members are able to raise questions and comment on individual statements.

If individuals feel that they do not wish to make a contribution they can refuse their turn by saying ''I pass''. It is essential that the leader helps to facilitate an atmosphere where group members are encouraged to participate. At the same time, they should feel that it is right for them not to contribute if they do not wish to do so at that time.

Small Groups (sometimes called Buzz Groups)

Work which is carried out in small groups of three or four members provides for individual views to be expressed and for people to get to know each other. Some individuals prefer to express their ideas in a small group rather than a large one. Small groups allow for greater involvement and use of existing knowledge, as well as a pooling of ideas.

When allocating tasks to small groups, it is essential that everyone should be absolutely clear that they understand the nature of the task. This may sound like stating the obvious, but in practice, small groups sometimes find they are doing something quite different from each other! It is helpful if the leader circulates among the small groups to check what they are doing.

It is an essential part of small group work that the findings of their activities are shared. One member of the small group is elected to report back on behalf of the others. Such a person is often referred to as a spokesperson (or reporter).

When reporting back, it may be necessary to ask each spokesperson in turn to report on some of their findings only. If one group is allowed to give all its feedback at once, it may pre-empt what the others have to say. It is better to take one or two points from one group, then move to the next group and so on, depending on the nature of the exercise.

Continuum (On the Line)

A continuum provides an opportunity for individuals to identify where their opinions place them between two extremes of an issue. For example, the two extremes could be:

(a)   'An individual is responsible for his/her own good health'

        and

(b)   'Good health is the government's responsiblity'

The group leader then explains these two extremes to the group. An imaginary line is 'drawn' from one side of the room to the other, usually down the centre. The extreme views can be displayed at either end of the 'line' on large sheets of paper or card.

An individual
is responsible for————————————————————————————————the government's
his/her own good health

Good health is
responsibility

The leader then asks group members to position themselves, one at a time, on the line somewhere between the two extremes where they feel that their current opinions would place them. As they stand on the line, each one says why she has taken up that position but discussion does not occur until all members are in place on the line. The leader then asks if all are happy with the position they have taken up; if not, they may move position if they wish. If a group member decides to change, she should give the reason for the move. There is much discussion as people move around the line and this can act as a trigger for further activities when the group re-forms.

In the programme, this activity has been adapted to help group members discuss their perceptions of weight. Although the extremes are given as 'Person A is very overweight' and 'Person B is very underweight' the principles used in carrying out the exercise are the same as those described above.

Course Ending

'Regrets and Appreciates' provides an opportunity for group members and the leader to share their feelings about the programme. Group members (and the leader) are asked to say one thing they have regretted (not enjoyed) about the course and one thing that they have appreciated (enjoyed). This activity is often conducted as a round, or it may be carried out informally: individuals speak as the opportunity arises. Such an activity is also a useful way to complete a course.

List of Activities

Session One

1.1 Introduction and warm-up activity
1.2 Why learn about healthy eating?
1.3 Healthy Eating card game
1.4 Name that Food!
1.5 Assignments: eating diary
             food labels

Session Two

2.1 The Name Game
2.2 Is it your choice?
2.3 Appraisal of food and drink diary
2.4 Find your way round a label
2.5 Assignment: hidden sugar in food

Session Three

3.1   Round: hidden sugar in food
3.2   Why less sugar?
3.3   A Day in the Life . . .
3.4   Going shopping
3.5   Changes
3.6   The Salt Picture

Session Four

4.1   Dietary Fibre: what it is and what it does
4.2   Mix and Match—a healthy role for fibre
4.3   Dietary fibre in your Food
4.4   Quiz—How many do you know?

Session Five

5.1   Fat—Where are You?
5.2   Fat—Who needs It?
5.3   Fatty Dip
5.4   Healthy Eating . . .?
5.5   Hints and Tips
5.6   Preparation for Group Project

Session Six

6.1   On the Line
6.2   Looking Back
6.3   Finalising group project arrangements
6.4   Food presentation

Session Seven

7.1   Group Project
7.2   Something New?
7.3   Regrets and Appreciates

SESSION ONE

Session One

Contents   Session Plan

Group Material:
  Healthy Eating Card Game
  Task Sheet: Name that Food!
  Food and Drink Diary
Leader's Material:
  How to Play the Healthy Eating Card Game
  Checklist: Name that Food!

Aids   Flip-chart/overhead projector and transparencies (OHP/Ts)
Felt-tip pens
Pens/pencils
Writing paper

Objectives   1   To enable group members to get to know each other.
2   To be aware of some of the reasons why healthy eating is important.
3   To clarify some of the misconceptions about food.
4   To introduce the use of a diary to monitor individual eating patterns.

Activity 1.1 is a warm-up activity (see section on participatory learning). Group leaders may wish to introduce an alternative warm-up activity if the group members are already known to each other.

The second activity (1.2) 'Why learn about healthy eating?' introduces the participatory learning methods used throughout the course. It helps individuals to know each other and promotes discussion about healthy eating.

The card game (Activity 1.3) is invaluable in building up the interaction process between group members. It helps group members to identify that they already have knowledge and opinions on which they are basing their current food choices. The questions were devised using the facts and fallacies which are often presented to dietitians and other professionals involved in nutrition education.

There is usually a demand from groups for information about reading food labels. Activity 1.4 'Name that Food!' is a light-hearted way to introduce reading and interpreting food labels to the group. Working through this exercise helps group members to realise what types of ingredients are present in processed food (this activity is followed up in Session Two). In the time between this session and the next one, group members should be encouraged to read food labels for themselves.

The final activity (1.5) in this session assigns a task to the group members which is to be completed before the next session. Each individual is asked to keep a diary in which she records the food and drink (kind and amount) personally consumed over a short period of time. The purpose of this activity is to help group members to assess objectively their own patterns of eating. As eating times may be irregular through shift-work, cultural patterns or family circumstances, traditional mealtimes are omitted from the record. At least three diary sheets will be needed for each group member (see activity 1.5).

Group members are asked to bring a food label to the next meeting of the group for use during that session.

SESSION PLAN

Activity number	Activity/time	Organisation, methods and content
1.1	INTRODUCTION AND WARM-UP ACTIVITY 10 minutes	(a) Leader welcomes group members and outlines domestic details and initial ground rules (b) Leader asks group members to introduce themselves to the group
1.2	WHY LEARN ABOUT HEALTHY EATING? 20 minutes	(a) Group forms into small groups of three or four (b) Leader asks groups to discuss briefly: i) why they wanted to come to the healthy eating course; ii) why they consider healthy eating to be important. Members of small groups should check they know each other's names before starting the exercise. Each group will need a spokesperson to report on the findings of their group. (c) Group re-forms to discuss findings. Leader receives feedback and records it on flip chart/OHT if wished.

Activity number	Activity/time	Organisation, methods and content
		(d) Leader briefly reviews points raised and explains the content of the programme.
1.3	HEALTHY EATING CARD GAME 45 minutes	(a) Leader explains how to play the card game.
		(b) Full group re-forms into small groups (maximum number is four).
		(c) Leader allocates one set of cards to each group and asks them to make a note, during play, of any points of interest to raise with the full group.
		(d) When all four sets of cards have been completed full group forms for discussion on points which have arisen during the game.
		(e) *Round*: 'One thing I have learned from playing the card game is . . .'
1.4	NAME THAT FOOD! 10 minutes	(a) Group work in pairs
		(b) Group leader distributes a copy of the quiz 'Name that Food!' and allows 5 minutes for all the foods to be identified.
		(c) Full group re-forms. One pair in turn reads out the possible identity of food number one. Leader checks identity from list. This process is repeated until all foods have been identified.

Activity number	Activity/time	Organisation, methods and content

1.5	ASSIGNMENTS
	5 minutes
	  Eating diary
	
	  Food Labels
		(a) Leader distributes food and drink diary sheets and asks group members to record all food and drink taken over a minimum of 3 days. More can be recorded if wished. (At least one day should be a weekend day.) The completed diaries should be brought to the next session. All diaries need to be dated. The information will be treated as confidential and need not be disclosed.
		(b) Group members to bring a food label or a food which has a label to the following session.

How to Play the Healthy Eating Card Game

1   It is essential that anyone using the Healthy Eating card game should try it out before using it with a group. This may be done with family, friends, or colleagues at work.

2   The game is made up of four sets of cards: each set consists of twelve question cards and twelve corresponding answer cards. Each card has a number which is shown on the top left hand corner of the card. Numbering of the sets is as follows:

Set one—numbers 1 to 12 inclusive

Set two—numbers 13 to 24 inclusive

Set three—numbers 25 to 36 inclusive

Set four—numbers 37 to 48 inclusive.

Before play starts it is important to check that the players are allocated the correct cards in each set. If the cards in the sets are wrong, the game is impossible to play properly.

3   The group forms into small groups of three or four (one complete pack of 48 cards is sufficient for sixteen people to play at any one time). Each small group sits in a circle; they are allocated one set of cards by the group leader.

4   Initially, the answer cards are put to one side (they will be used as a resource later in the game). One player deals out the cards to the others—each player will have three or four cards depending on the number of players in the small group.

5   The player who has the card with the lowest number in the top left hand corner starts to play. He reads out the question on the card and then chooses what he considers to be the right answer from the choices given on the card. At this stage, it should be the responsibility of the player to provide an answer. (If he does not know the answer, he can either make a guess or the group could help on some occasions. If the group were to discuss every answer the game would take too long to play.)

An example is given below:

Question

Card Number ———— Q.11 Brown eggs are better for health than white ones:

Possible answers

a)   True   3 — Alternative card

b)   False   12 — numbers for follow-on by next player

The player says "Brown eggs are better for health than white ones. I think that statement is false—who has card number 12?". The player who has card number 12 then reads out her question and gives the answer, followed by the number of the next card. The player who has that card reads out the next question, and so on, until all the cards have been played. (Sometimes a player will have been dealt two consecutive cards but this does not matter—the game continues and all players will have their turn).

6   As players answer the question cards these should be placed face upwards in a circle on a table or the floor (as there are twelve cards they can be placed in the same position as the numbers on a clock face).

7   If all the answers are correct, all the players will be left without cards in their hands. The number which corresponds to the correct answer on the last card played must lead to the number in the top left hand corner on the first card played. If the numbers do not correspond or the players have cards left in their hands then one or more of the questions has been answered incorrectly.

In order to find out where they have made mistakes, the group goes back over the answers, and the discussion then takes place to find out which questions were answered correctly and which may be wrong. The group then consults the appropriate answer card(s) and replays the set until all the answers are correct and the numbers on the last and first cards to be played correspond.

8   The game is over when all four sets have been played by each small group.

9   As the game is in progress, group members should write down points they are not sure of or anything else they would like to raise in discussion when the full group re-forms.

10   It will also be beneficial if group members go through the questions and answers at the end of each set. Often the right answer is given, but the group members do not know the reason why a particular answer is correct. There is much information to be gained from the answer cards which may be lost if this final brief exercise is not carried out.

The Healthy Eating card game can also be used as a quiz—it can also be used for introducing healthy eating to any group as it encourages group discussion which will generate interest.

(Patent No. 1601216)

HEALTHY EATING CARD GAME

Q.1 Fried foods absorb some of the fat (or oil) in which they are cooked:

a) True   7
b) False   4

Q.2 Meat is essential for health:

a) True   11
b) False   8

Q.3 You need less food as you get older:

a) True   10
b) False   6

Q.4 Which vitamin is associated with sunshine:

a) Vitamin C?   2
b) Vitamin D?   5

Q.5 All tinned fruit is preserved in sugar syrup:

a) True   8
b) False   2

Q.6 Canned minestrone soup is a good substitute for a meal:

a) True   7
b) False   1

Q.7 Honey is good for you:

a) True   5
b) False   4

Q.8 Whilst on a weight-reducing diet, bread and potatoes should be excluded from your diet:

a) True   12
b) False   11

Q.9 In which of the following foods would you find dietary fibre:

a) Meat?   10
b) Peas?   3

Q.10 Fat is present in:

a) Victoria sandwich cake   6
b) Jacket potato   1

Q.11 Brown eggs are better for health than white ones:

a) True 9
b) False 12

Q.12 Chicken has a lower fat content than many other meats:

a) True 9
b) False 3

Q.13 Water is present in all foods. Which one of the following foods has the most water:

a) Cabbage? 15
b) Butter? 23

Q.14 People who have big bones are always overweight:

a) True 21
b) False 18

Q.15 Diabetic jam is low in calories:

a) True 14
b) False 23

Q.16 All powdered milks are low in fat:

a) True 13
b) False 19

Q.17 Which fruit has the higher content of Vitamin C

a) An apple? 20
b) A grapefruit? 22

Q.18 All fruit yoghurts are low in fat and sugar.

a) True 17
b) False 21

Q.19 Sugar is necessary for energy:

a) True 15
b) False 13

Q.20 Is it true that crinkle-cut chips absorb more fat than straight sided chips:

a) Yes? 24
b) No? 16

Q.21 Foods, particularly those with a high sugar
content, are more likely to cause tooth decay
if eaten:

a) Immediately before meals   22
b) Between meals   17

Q.22 A high-fibre diet will help to relieve constipation:

a) True   20
b) False   24

Q.23 Baked beans are high in fibre:

a) True   14
b) False   18

Q.24 Cheaper cuts of meat can be as good as the
expensive ones:

a) True   16
b) False   19

Q.25 The best way of increasing fibre in the diet
is:

a) Adding bran to the food   33
b) Eating more foods which are naturally
high in fibre   27

Q.26 When you buy prepacked food you can
identify the main ingredient in the product
by knowing it is:

a) First on the list of ingredients 36
b) Last on the list of ingredients   34

Q.27 Vitamin pills are essential for a healthy diet:

a) True   31
b) False   33

Q.28 Which of the following is not another form
of sugar?

a) Glucose syrup   25
b) Saccharine   35

Q.29 Alcohol can be a nourishing replacement for
a midday meal as a liquid lunch:

a) True   30
b) False   32

Q.30 Sauna baths help you to lose weight:

a) True   35
b) False   28

Q.31 One way of reducing the amount of sugar in the diet is to use:

a) Low-calorie orange drink   26
b) Lemonade   36

Q.32 Which of the following foods is likely to contain sugar:

a) Tomato salad?   30
b) Tomato ketchup?   28

Q.33 A high-fat diet is linked with:

a) Lung cancer   36
b) Coronary heart disease   31

Q.34 Which one of the following contains the highest amount of dietary fibre:

a) One slice of white bread?   32
b) One slice of wholemeal bread?   29

Q.35 Cooking green vegetables for a long time damages their food value:

a) True   25
b) False   27

Q.36 Eating salads is the only way to lose weight:

a) True   29
b) False   34

Q.37 An apple a day keeps the doctor away:

a) True   45
b) False   40

Q.38 A diet which is high in fibre is more likely to reduce the incidence of:

a) Bowel disorders   43
b) Cirrhosis of the liver   47

Q.39 Oil is less fattening than lard or butter:

a) True   42
b) False   46

Q.40 Low-fat spreads are lower in calories than butter or margarine because the low-fat spreads have:

a) A higher water content   45
b) A higher starch content   38

Q.41 Grapefruit 'magics away' fat:

    a) True   40
    b) False   37

Q.42 Which one of the following foods has a low salt content:

    a) Bacon?   44
    b) Fresh cod?   48

Q.43 Fat can be absorbed into the body through the skin:

    a) True   39
    b) False   47

Q.44 A diet high in salt may be associated with high blood pressure (hypertension):

    a) True   41
    b) False   37

Q.45 If you eat more food than your body uses, the excess energy is stored as body fat:

    a) True   38
    b) False   43

Q.46 Cake, biscuits and pastries are an essential part of a healthy diet:

    a) True   48
    b) False   42

Q.47 One hundred grams (one small packet) of boiled sweets can contain:

    a) 9 teaspoons of sugar   46
    b) 18 teaspoons of sugar   39

Q.48 In the eighteenth century in Britain the amount of sugar consumed was about 2 kg (about 4 lb) per head per year. It is now estimated to be:

    a) 38 kg (84 lb)/head/year   44
    b) 54 kg (124 lb)/head/year   41

A.1   Fried foods do absorb some of the fat in which they are cooked. Cooking the food by grilling, baking, boiling, poaching or steaming will not increase the fat content of the food.

     The statement is therefore TRUE.
     Move on to card number 7.

A.2   A meal without meat can still be nourishing. You can get all the protein and nutrients you need from other foods, so meat need not necessarily be included in a healthy diet.

     The statement is therefore FALSE.
     Move on to card number 8.

A.3   As people get older they become less active and require less energy from food, but still need adequate amounts of all nutrients. A good varied diet with fewer foods that are high in sugar and/or high in fat will help to provide a healthy diet for the elderly.

     The statement is therefore TRUE.
     Move on to card number 10.

A.4   Vitamin D is produced in the body as a result of the exposure of skin to sunlight.

     The answer is therefore (b).
     Move on to card number 5.

A.5   Several food manufacturers produce fruit that is tinned in natural juices.

     The statement is therefore FALSE.
     Move on to card number 2.

A.6   Most tinned or packet soups have little food value and are therefore not a good substitute for a meal. Make lentil soup or add cheese, milk, meat or vegetables to a soup to improve its food value.

     The statement is therefore FALSE.
     Move on to card number 1.

A.7   Honey is mainly sugar. Despite its special reputation it has no properties as a health-giving food.

     The statement is therefore FALSE.
     Move on to card number 4.

A.8   Bread and potatoes can form a valuable part of a weight-reducing diet. Both types of food, if eaten with little or no added fat, are very satisfying without having a high energy value.

     The statement is therefore FALSE.
     Move on to card number 11.

A.9   Dietary fibre is found only in foods of plant origin. It is the substance which forms the cell walls and gives the rigid structure to all plants.

     The answer is therefore (b).
     Move on to card number 3.

A.10   Fat is present in a Victoria sandwich cake in the form of butter or margarine, depending on the recipe, and also in the egg yolks. Potatoes do not contain fat.

     The answer is therefore (a).
     Move on to card number 6.

A.11 The food value of brown eggs is just the same as that of white eggs.

The statement is therefore FALSE.
Move on to card number 12.

A.12 Chicken *is* lower in fat than many other meats, and can make a useful contribution to a healthy diet.

The statement is therefore TRUE.
Move on to card number 9.

A.13 Many vegetables have a high water content, approximately 70–90% water. This high water content contributes to their low energy value as water does not provide energy.

The answer is therefore (a).
Move on to card number 15.

A.14 The size of bones does make a difference to the weight of a person, but having big bones does not necessarily mean that a person will be overweight.

The statement is therefore FALSE.
Move on to card number 18.

A.15 Many proprietary diabetic foods, including jam, are sweetened by agents other than sugar which are just as high in calories.

The statement is therefore FALSE.
Move on to card number 23.

A.16 Some powdered milks are simply dried skimmed milk and are therefore low in fat. Others are skimmed milk powder with added vegetable fat. Read the label to determine what you are buying.

The statement is therefore FALSE.
Move on to card number 19.

A.17 Grapefruit and other citrus fruits, eg. oranges and lemons, are among the richest common sources of vitamin C. Apples do contain vitamin C but not in such high concentration.

The answer is therefore (b).
Move on to card number 22.

A.18 Not all yoghurts are low in fat and/or sugar. The information on the label will help you to find out about the fat and sugar content of a yoghurt.

The statement is therefore FALSE.
Move on to card number 21.

A.19 Sugar does provide energy but so do all the other foods we eat. Sugar and many of its by-products, such as golden syrup, provide little food value and are not necessary to keep us healthy or provide us with energy.

The statement is therefore FALSE.
Move on to card number 13.

A.20 Crinkle-cut chips have a greater surface area in contact with the fat, so more fat is absorbed.

The answer is therefore YES.
Move on to card number 24.

A.21 Food and drink containing added sugar are particularly likely to cause tooth decay if consumed between meals.

The answer is therefore (b).
Move on to card number 17.

A.22 As fibre passes through the digestive system it absorbs fluid. This softens and increases the bulk of the stools so that they are more easily passed, thus helping to relieve constipation.

The statement is therefore TRUE.
Move on to card number 20.

A.23 All pulses (eg. peas, beans and lentils) are high in fibre. Baked beans are prepared from haricot beans, a member of the pulse family, and therefore have a high fibre content.

The statement is therefore TRUE.
Move on to card number 14.

A.24 Cheaper cuts of meat tend to be more fatty than the more expensive, leaner cuts. By trimming all excess fat and removing liquid fat from gravies, casseroles and stews, the cheaper cuts of meat compare favourably with the more expensive ones. Many people eat more meat than they need. Some of the meat in dishes such as stews and casseroles could be replaced by beans, eg. red kidney beans or butter beans.

The statement is therefore TRUE.
Move on to card number 16.

A.25 It is preferable to increase the fibre intake by eating more foods which are naturally high in fibre, eg. wholemeal bread and whole grain cereals, rather than adding bran to a refined diet.

The answer is therefore (b).
Move on to card number 27.

A.26 Ingredients have to be listed in order of quantity. The main ingredient is therefore listed first. The further the ingredient down the list, the less there will be of it in the food.

The answer is therefore (a).
Move on to card number 36.

A.27 If you are eating a healthy diet with a wide variety of foods, you should get all the vitamins you need without supplementing it with vitamin pills.

The statement is therefore FALSE.
Move on to card number 33.

A.28 Saccharine is an artificial sweetener—it does not contain sugar. Sugar comes in a variety of forms such as glucose, glucose syrup, dextrose and maltose.

The answer is therefore (b).
Move on to card number 35.

A.29 Alcoholic drinks have little nutritive value and therefore cannot be used to replace any meal. They are high in calories and if they are used frequently to replace food, a person can become overweight but still be malnourished.

The statement is therefore FALSE.
Move on to card number 32.

A.30 In sauna baths where the temperature is very high, the body will sweat to try and cool itself; this fluid loss is largely water, not fat. A cup of tea or a long cool drink will soon replace this loss.

The statement is therefore FALSE.
Move on to card number 28.

A.31 In low-calorie drinks the sugar (or much of the sugar) is replaced by artificial sweeteners. This reduces the calorie content and therefore the energy value. Lemonade contains a high proportion of sugar.

The answer is therefore (a).
Move on to card number 26.

A.32 Many manufactured or processed foods contain sugar; this is indicated on the food labels.

The answer is therefore (b).
Move on to card number 30.

A.33 A high-fat diet is linked with coronary heart disease.

The answer is therefore (b).
Move on to card number 31.

A.34 Wholemeal bread is made from flour containing the whole of the wheat grain. Part of the wheat grain is removed in the refining process used to produce brown and white flours. This reduces the fibre value, especially of white flour and therefore of white bread.

Wholemeal bread contains 8.5% fibre.
White bread contains 2.5% fibre.

The answer is therefore (b).
Move on to card number 29.

A.35 Some of the nutritive value of vegetables, especially green leafy vegetables, is readily destroyed by overcooking. To preserve the maximum food value of vegetables, it is wise to cook for the minimum amount of time, or where possible to eat raw.

The statement is therefore TRUE.
Move on to card number 25.

A.36 Although salads are most useful in a weight-reducing diet, many other suitable foods can be included in such a diet to give variety. Many recipes, including those for salads, are available to make weight loss more interesting.

The statement is therefore FALSE.
Move on to card number 34.

A.37 Apples can form a useful part of a healthy diet, but unfortunately are not a guarantee that the doctor will stay away!

The statement is therefore FALSE.
Move on to card number 40.

A.38 There is strong evidence that a low-fibre diet is linked with bowel disorders such as constipation. Fibre in the diet can provide some protection against such disorders.

The answer is therefore (a).
Move on to card number 43.

A.39 Oils are fats which are liquid at room temperature. As with all fats, they have a high energy value.

The statement is therefore FALSE.
Move on to card number 46.

A.40 Low-fat spreads are a blend of vegetable oils and water. They contain half the fat of either butter or margarine.

The answer is therefore (a).
Move on to card number 45.

A.41 This statement is false—grapefruit has no magical properties. It is often included in weight-reducing diets because it has a low energy value.

    The statement is therefore FALSE.
Move on to card number 37.

A.42 Many processed foods are high in salt (sodium chloride) as it acts as a useful preservative. Most fresh foods are poor sources of salt.

    The answer is therefore (b).
Move on to card number 48.

A.43 Some people who work with food (eg. in a fish and chip shop) believe that their weight problems are due to fat being absorbed through their skin. It is much more likely that tasting the food is the cause of the problem! Fat which comes into contact with the skin can only penetrate the outer layers and will not be utilized by the body.

    The answer is therefore FALSE.
Move on to card number 47.

A.44 Most people eat more salt than is needed by the body. Many experts believe that a diet which has a high salt content may be linked with high blood pressure.

    The statement is therefore TRUE.
Move on to card number 41.

A.45 The statement is TRUE!.
Move on to card number 38.

A.46 The majority of cakes, biscuits and pastries are high in fat and sugar and are not essential as part of a healthy diet.

    The statement is therefore FALSE.
Move on to card number 42.

A.47 One hundred grams (one small packet) of boiled sweets can contain 18 teaspoons of sugar.

    The answer is therefore (b).
Move on to card number 39.

A.48 The amount of sugar consumed in Britain has dramatically increased since the eighteenth century to a peak of 54 kg/head/year in 1974, gradually declining to an estimated value of 38 kg/head/year (1980 figure provided by the Ministry of Agriculture, Fisheries and Food).

    The answer is therefore (a).
Move on to card number 44.

Task Sheet: Name that Food!

The foods listed below have no names . . . they are the ingredients of various packaged foods which are everyday items: *how many of them can you name?*

1   Cheese, reconstituted skimmed milk powder, butter, emulsifying salts (E339, E450C), whey powder, salt.

2   Maltodextrin, food starch, vegetable fat, flavourings, hydrolysed protein, tomato powder, salt, sugar, colours (E150, E124), dried oxtail, dried beef, beef fat, flavour enhancer (monosodium glutamate), citric acid (E330) and antioxidant (E320/E321).

3   Pork, chicken, water, beef, vegetable protein, dry skimmed milk, salt, spices, sodium tripolyphosphate (E450C), antioxidant: ascorbic acid, preservative: sodium nitrate.

4   Sugar, invert sugar syrup, glucose syrup, water, gelatine, citric acid, acetic acid, lemon juice, essential oil of lemon, flavouring, acidity regulator (sodium citrate), artificial sweetener (sodium saccharin), colours (E102, E110).

5   Water, glucose syrup, oranges, citric acid, stabiliser, preservatives, artificial sweetener (saccharin), colours, flavouring.

6   Starch, wheat flour, colour (E150), soya flour, treacle, dried yeast, hydrolysed vegetable protein, flavour enhancer (monosodium glutamate), dried onion, lactose, dried carrot, flavouring, vegetable fat, spices.

7   Starch, salt, colours (E102, E110, E127), flavourings.

8   Skimmed milk, vegetable fat, food starch, emulsifiers, sugar, edible gum, flavouring.

9   Soya protein mince (defatted soya flour, caramel, iron sulphate, thiamine, riboflavin, vitamin B12), starch, fat, onion, hydrolysed protein, lactose, salt, tomato, monosodium glutamate, yeast extract, sodium caseinate, beef, spices, emulsifier.

10 Sugar, wheat flour, water, cherries, vegetable fat (with antioxidant E321), dried glucose syrup, modified starch, skimmed milk powder, cheese powder, gelling agents (E327, E339, E450), sodium caseinate, emulsifier (E472B), stabiliser (E401), salt, fumaric acid, citric acid (E330), flavourings, preservative (E211), colours (E102, E122, E124, E142, E151).

Checklist: Name that Food!

1   Cheese spread

2   Oxtail soup (instant packet soup)

3   Hot dog sausages

4   Lemon jelly

5   Orange drink

6   Gravy powder

7   Custard powder

8   Dessert topping

9   Soya mince with onion

10   Cherry cheesecake mix

Food and Drink Diary   **Date** _____

TIME	WHAT WAS EATEN (INCLUDING DRINKS)

SESSION TWO

Session Two

Contents   Session Plan

Group Material:
  Task Sheet: Appraisal of Food and Drink Diary
  Task Sheet: Find Your Way Round a Label (with diagram*)
Leader's Material:
  Checklist: Is It Your Choice?
  Background Information: Find Your Way Round a Label

Aids   Flip-chart/OHP/Ts
Felt-tip pens
Pens/pencils
Envelopes for food assessment diaries
Food labels—in case group members forget to bring their own

Objectives 1 To enable the group to get to know each other's names.
          2 To identify some of the main reasons which influence the group members' choice of food.
          3 To make an appraisal of the food and drink diary completed between the two sessions.
          4 To find out the type of information which is contained on food labels.
          5 To encourage group members to read food labels before Session Three.

As the group members may have started meeting especially for the course the leader may find it useful to start with a simple warm-up game (Activity 2.1). The example given in the plan is called the 'Name Game'. This particular exercise generates some fun, especially if the group leader is prepared to go last and say everyone's name in the circle. Other warm-up games may be more appropriate if the group members know each other well.

The second exercise (Activity 2.2) 'Is it your choice?' helps the group to understand the large number of factors which influence the food choices individuals make. The group will already be aware of some of these, but the brainstorn will generate numerous ideas, some of which will not have been realised by individuals.

In the context of this basic programme, the time is too limited to spend on developing work on food choices. However, this activity could be useful for starting discussions on family nutrition, women's roles, the availability of healthy food in cafés and restaurants, weight watching, and so on.

'Appraising your food and drink diary' (Activity 2.3) is carried out using the diary completed between Sessions One and Two. The leader will need to stress that

---

*The label interpretation diagram may need to be photocopied or drawn on a flip-chart or OHP, depending on the facilities which are available.

completing the appraisal sheet is not a test of knowledge and that group members will review the appraisal in a later session. Alternatively, the diary and appraisal sheet may be referred to at appropriate stages throughout the course.

Twenty minutes is allowed for group members to work on the appraisal of their eating patterns and the food they eat. During this period group members may wish to share information with other group members and/or the leader. The written information given remains confidential. The diary and appraisal sheet are put into an envelope, sealed, and retained by the group leader until the end of the course (it will be necessary for names to be written on the outside of the envelopes). Anyone who forgets his diary, or loses it, may complete the appraisal sheet by recalling all the food and drink that he consumed during the previous twenty-four hours.

The remainder of the session is concerned with finding out the kind of information which may be obtained from food labels (Activity 2.4). Food labelling is a topic which always generates much discussion, and the activities also act as an introduction to hidden fat, sugar and salt.

The assignment 'Hidden sugar in foods' (Activity 2.5) forms a link between the activities in this session and those of Session Three which focus on the presence of sugar in foods.

SESSION PLAN

Activity number	Activity/time	Organisation, methods and content
2.1	THE NAME GAME 10 minutes	(a) Leader explains the purpose of a warm-up game and explains how to play the 'Name Game'. (b) Group plays the 'Name Game'.
2.2	IS IT YOUR CHOICE? 15 minutes	(a) Leader explains that there are a large number of factors which influence what people eat, eg. cost, availability, appearance. (b) *Brainstorm*: the factors which influence what you eat. Leader writes suggestions on flip-chart/OHT. (c) As a full group discuss the points raised.

Activity number	Activity/time	Organisation, methods and content

2.3	APPRAISAL OF FOOD AND DRINK DIARY
	20 minutes
		(a) Leader distributes appraisal sheets to group and asks each member to complete them using their eating diaries completed between Sessions One and Two.
		(b) Leader explains that:
		   (i) if any help is required this may be obtained by talking to other group members or the leader;
		   (ii) the information is confidential;
		   (iii) the appraisal will be required later in the course, hence the need for envelopes.

2.4	FIND YOUR WAY ROUND A LABEL 40 minutes	(a) Using the label interpretation diagram, leader describes the key information which must be shown on prepacked food. (b) Group forms into pairs. Leader ensures that each group has a variety of labels or foods which have a label on the packaging. (c) Leader hands out the question sheets 'Find your way round a label'. (d) Leader provides information as required. (e) When the question sheets have been completed leader discusses points raised with full group.

Activity number	Activity/time	Organisation, methods and content
2.5	ASSIGNMENT: HIDDEN SUGAR IN FOOD 5 minutes	(a) Leader explains that sugar is often contained in foods which are not considered to be very sweet or to have sugar in the ingredients. (b) Leader asks the members to look at labels before the next session and to find at least one food which contains 'hidden sugar'. A discussion on the group's findings will open Session Three.

Checklist: Is It Your Choice?

Reasons for Choosing and Eating Food

Do people really have a free choice when they come to select their food? This exercise helps group members to consider the factors which contribute to their choice of food. Individual group members will attach different degrees of importance to each factor.

The following list gives some indication of the factors influencing food choice which may be identified by the group:

Health
Hunger
Variety
To suit needs of individual: age, sex, work
Diet: eg. diabetic, vegetarian, slimming
Allergies
Religion/culture/beliefs
Life style
Family habits, eg. chips always go with fish
Likes and dislikes—of self, of family, of those sharing meal
To be sociable
The occasion, eg. family meal, celebration, whether eating at home or away
Whether the food was chosen by self, or presented by others
Availability in shops
Season
Availability of freezer/microwave
Income
Price of individual foods
The need to use up leftovers
Convenience
Preparation time
Appearance of foods
Texture
Odour of food
Childhood associations
Comfort
Boredom
Advertising

Task Sheet: Appraising your Food and Drink Diary

The following questions are designed to help you to become more aware of your current eating patterns. You will find it helpful to use your diary as you work through the questions. When you get to the end write your name on the envelope provided, put your diary and appraisal sheet with it and hand it to the group leader. The information which you have disclosed will be treated as confidential.

1   On average, how many times did you eat during the day?

2   For how many meals did *you* choose what you ate?

3   Look through your eating diary and list all the foods that you think contain sugar.

4   Using one day of your eating diary list the foods which you think are high in fibre (roughage).

5   Decide which foods in your eating diary contain fat. Using one day of your eating diary list those foods you think may be high in fat.

6 List any foods to which you normally add salt.

7 List the food choices you made which you think are in line with current nutritional recommendations.

8 Have you made any major changes in your eating patterns over the last year? If so, please say what they are.

9 Are there any changes you feel you would like to make in your present eating pattern?

10 Are there any comments you would like to make about your eating patterns and choice of food?

FIND YOUR WAY ROUND A LABEL

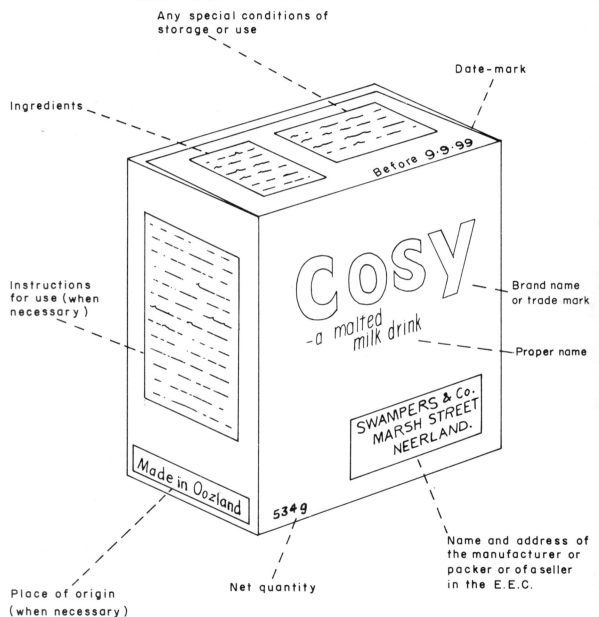

This diagram illustrates the information which must be shown on pre-packed food.

Task Sheet: Find your Way Round a Label

1   What is the name of the food? Does it have a trademark?

2   What is the main ingredient?

3   Where does the food's main flavour come from?

4   Have any additives been used?

5   Is there a date-mark?

6   What is the net quantity of the food?

7   Does the label inform you of the best way to store the food?

8   Are any claims made about the food, eg. is it suitable for slimmers or does it contain certain vitamins? If the answer is yes, the claim should be backed up with supporting information on the label. See if you can find it.

9   Who would you contact if you required further information about the food?

10   Is the place of origin of the food stated on the label?

Background Information: Find Your Way Round a Label

The group members will carry out this task by referring to a variety of food labels. The following comments will give guidance on how each question might be answered.

Q1   What is the name of the food? Does it also have a brand name or trademark?

A1   This may sound a simple question, but it is often not realised that a food is frequently known by the brand name or a trademark rather than its proper name. The following example can be used to help clarify this point:

A malted milk drink is called 'Cosy'. A purchaser in a shop will ask for 'Cosy'—Cosy is its brand or trade name. Its proper name (or the name of the food) is 'malted milk drink'—the name which helps to describe to customers what kind of food they are buying.

Some of the names are prescribed by law and describe exactly what the food is, for instance, orange squash, wholemeal bread. Others have a customary name, ie. the name a food is traditionally known by, such as fish fingers, Battenburg cake.

Those foods which do not have a legally prescribed or a customary name will have a descriptive name, ie. one which accurately describes the food, eg. yeast extract.

The brand name or trade name should be quite distinct from the name of the food.

Q2   What is the main ingredient?

A2   The ingredients are listed in descending order of weight: the main ingredient is the one listed first.

Q3   Where does the food's main flavour come from—is it from the food itself or from added flavouring?

A3   The following will help to answer this question:
Example: Food label: Raspberry Yoghurt
(a)   If the flavouring comes from the fruit, the label will carry the words 'raspberry' or 'raspberry flavoured'. If the wording is 'raspberry flavour' yoghurt the main flavour would be obtained from sources other than the fruit. This principle applies to foods other than yoghurts.

44

(b)   The food pictured on the label must be that from which the flavour is mainly or wholly derived.

(c)   The list of ingredients will also provide further information.

In the example given the flavour came from the fruit itself.

Q4   Have any additives been used?

A4   Check the list of ingredients. An additive will be listed by the main function it performs, eg. anticaking agent, flavour enhancer, followed by its chemical name or its serial number, eg. E number or simply a number (many additives have non-E numbers).

Q5   Is there a datemark?

A5   Most prepacked foods will have a date-mark. One exception is foods which will last for more than 18 months. The date-mark indicates how long the food will keep, if stored properly, and still remain of good quality. Look for the phrases: 'Best before', 'Best before end', 'Sell by'.

Q6   What is the net quantity of the food?

A6   The net quantity of the food will be shown in metric units. If the label shows the **e** mark this signifies that the goods are packed in accordance with the relevant EEC directive. It may only be used when the quantity of the goods are within the range 5 g – 10 kg (5 ml – 10 l).

Q7   Does the label inform you of the best way to store the food?

A7   Any special instructions for storage will be given. The date-marks are based on the assumption that the food will be stored properly.

Q8   Are any claims made about the food, eg. suitable for slimmers or contains certain vitamins? If yes, the claim should be backed up with supporting information.

A8   A claim about the food cannot be made unless the food can fulfil the claim, and the details of how it does this are marked on the label.

Q9   Who would you contact if you required further information about the food?

A9   The name and address of the manufacturer, packer or seller will be on the label. They should be able to help you with any further information you may require regarding the food.

Q10   Is the place of origin of the food stated on the label?

A10   The place of origin of the food should be stated on the label, because without it the purchaser might be misled as to its real origin.

SESSION THREE

Session Three

Contents   Session Plan

Group Material:
    Task Sheet: 'A Day in the Life . . .' Case Study
    Task Sheet: The Salt Picture
Leader's Material:
    Background Information:
      Why Less Sugar?
      The Salt Picture
Checklist: 'A Day in the Life . . .'
Checklist: 'Going Shopping'
Checklist: The Salt Picture

Aids   Flip-chart/OHP/Ts
Felt-tip pens
Pens/pencils
Writing paper

Objectives
1 To identify 'hidden sugar' in processed and packaged foods.
2 To identify reasons for reducing sugar.
3 To calculate the total amount of sugar in a case study.
4 To identify alternatives to high sugar foods.
5 To be aware of foods which are high in salt.
6 To know ways of reducing salt in the diet.

The opening round (Activity 3.1) provides a link with the activities on food labelling from the previous session. It highlights the use of 'hidden sugar' in packaged and processed foods. There are usually a number of surprises at the wide variety of such foods which contain sugar.

'Why Less Sugar?' (Activity 3.2) enables the group to discuss why they think that sugar consumption in the diet should be reduced. The ideas generated by the group can be clarified at the end of the exercise.

The activities which follow help group members to relate their knowledge of sugar to everyday situations. 'A Day in the Life . . .' (Activity 3.3) is a case study which enables group members to quantify the amount of sugar consumed in a fictitious day's food intake.

To make the exercise more meaningful, the quantities of sugar are given in teaspoons rather than in grams. It is also a useful exercise for the leader to illustrate the quantity of sugar consumed by demonstrating the number of teaspoons of sugar present in the case study. There are 39 teaspoons of sugar so a large receptacle is needed. If the amount of sugar is weighed, this will help to reinforce the points made in the session.

'Going Shopping' (Activity 3.4) enables the group to think how they can relate the information gained to their own shopping expeditions.

'Changes' (Activity 3.5) is an activity which uses sugar to illustrate the principle that changes which are in line with the NACNE Report recommendations are possible in the context of an individual's own eating pattern.

The salt picture explores the various aspects of the presence of salt in the daily food intake. For a complete picture the following points are raised:

(a) the possible relationship between salt and blood pressure;
(b) situations where salt is added to food;
(c) the content of salt in fresh and processed foods;
(d) alternatives to salt.

SESSION PLAN

Activity number	Activity/time	Organisation, methods and content
3.1	ROUND: HIDDEN SUGAR IN FOODS 10 minutes	(a) Each individual identifies a food which he has found contains 'hidden sugar'. (b) Leader asks the group what they have learned from this exercise. (c) Leader asks the group how they have been able to use the information from the previous session on food labelling.
3.2	WHY LESS SUGAR? 15 minutes	(a) Group works in small groups of three or four. (b) Leader explains that the current nutritional recommendations suggest that our sugar consumption should be reduced. (c) Each sub-group discusses this recommendation and records the reason why they think the recommendation has been made. (d) Sub-groups report back to full group. Discuss the results of the exercise.

Activity number	Activity/time	Organisation, methods and content
3.3	A DAY IN THE LIFE . . . 15 minutes	(a) Group works in pairs. (b) Leader hands out case study task sheets and guide and asks pairs to work out the total amount of sugar consumed in the case study. (c) As a full group, discuss the results of the exercise. (d) Leader demonstrates the amount of sugar in a variety of foods using the examples in the case study.
3.4	GOING SHOPPING 15 minutes	(a) Group works in pairs. (b) Leader asks group to imagine that they are out shopping with a friend. Each pair to decide on two ways of helping their friend to buy an alternative to a high-sugar food, eg. to buy fruit canned in natural juice rather than sugar syrup. (c) Full group reforms to share ideas.
3.5	CHANGES 10 minutes	(a) Leader asks full group for ways of reducing the sugar content in the case study 'A Day in the Life . . .'. Leader records suggestions appropriately. (b) Discuss as full group.

Activity number	Activity/time	Organisation, methods and content
3.6	THE SALT PICTURE 25 minutes	(a) Leader displays the following statement: ''Most of us eat far more salt than we need. Some experts believe that this intake of salt may be putting up the nation's blood pressure'' (Beating Heart Disease, Health Education Council 21/82). Leader explains this statement. (b) Group works in 4 small groups; each sub-group is handed a different task from 'The Salt Picture' as described in the accompanying notes. (c) When task is completed, full group re-forms. Each sub-group reports back on findings in order of the numbers written on their task sheets. (d) Leader clarifies information and completes picture where necessary. (e) Leader asks the group what they have learned from doing this exercise.

Background Information: Why Less Sugar?

The NACNE Report estimates that the consumption of sugar should be reduced from its current level of 38 kg per person per year to 20 kg per person per year. This represents a drop in consumption of about 50%.

Sugar comes in a variety of forms. The most common of these is white sugar which is added to tea and coffee or used in baking. This particular form of sugar is called sucrose. Food labels often indicate the presence of other sugars. These include glucose, glucose syrup, fructose, maltose, honey, molasses and brown sugar. Brown sugar, coloured sugar crystals and cube sugar are all different forms of sucrose.

It is the foods which contain these added sugars, as listed above, which should be reduced, rather than foods which contain natural sugars, eg. fruit. The latter are useful sources of other nutrients and make a valuable contribution to a healthy diet.

The following points need to be considered when discussing why sugar levels need to be reduced:

1. Sugar provides calories, or energy only; it has no other nutritional value. Much better alternative sources of energy are available from foods which provide other nutrients as well as energy, eg. unrefined foods: wholemeal bread, whole grain cereals.

2. Foods which have a high sugar content may displace other foods which are more nutritious.

3. Sugar and/or sugary food can lead to tooth decay, especially if consumed between meals.

4. As sugar is a concentrated form of energy, it can contribute to the problem of being overweight. This, in itself, is associated with other health problems such as heart disease and diabetes mellitus.

Task Sheet: 'A Day in the Life . . .' Case Study and Guide

The task sheet opposite shows the amount and kind of food and drink which someone might consume in one day. Some of the sugar taken during the day is added by the person . . . some of it was already present in the food. A guide to the amount of sugar in the foods consumed in the case study is given in the table below.

Work out the total amount of sugar (it's all in teaspoons) in the day's food and drink intake. To make it easy, write the amount of sugar for each item in the empty column marked 'teaspoons of sugar' on the chart shown and then add them up at the end.

A Guide to the Amount of Sugar in the Foods Mentioned in 'A Day in the Life . . .' Task Sheet

Food	Amount	Teaspoons of sugar
Cornflakes	1 bowl	½
Ginger nuts	1 biscuit	1
Sweet pickle	3 teaspoons	1
Fruit pie	1 individual	6
Milk chocolate	1 small bar	3½
Tomato ketchup	6 teaspoons	1½
Processed peas	1 portion	½
Fruit, canned in syrup	1 small can	5
Rice pudding, canned	1 can	5
Cola	1 can	7
Digestive biscuit	1 biscuit	½

Time	What was eaten (including drinks)	Teaspoons of sugar
8.30 am	Cornflakes (1 bowl) with milk and 2 teaspoons of sugar. 2 cups of tea with 1 teaspoon of sugar per cup.	
11.00 am	1 cup of coffee with 1 teaspoon of sugar. 2 ginger nuts.	
12.30 pm	Sandwiches made from 4 slices bread, cheese and 6 teaspoons mixed pickle. Packet of crisps. Individual apple pie. 1 cup of coffee with 1 teaspoon of sugar.	
3.00 pm	1 cup of tea with 1 teaspoon of sugar. 1 small bar milk chocolate.	
4.00 pm	1 cup of tea with 1 teaspoon of sugar.	
6.00 pm	Fish and chips. Tomato ketchup—6 teaspoons. 1 portion processed peas. ½ small tin fruit. ½ small tin rice pudding. Coffee with 1 teaspoon sugar.	
7.30 pm	Cola—1 tin.	
10.00 pm	1 cup of coffee with 1 teaspoon of sugar. 2 digestive biscuits.	
	Total	

Checklist: Ways of Reducing Sugar in the Case Study 'A Day in the Life . . .'

Food with a high sugar content	Alternatives with a lower sugar content
Sugar added to breakfast cereal and drinks	reduce amount used cut it out altogether substitute an artificial sweetener
Biscuits	use less sweet variety substitute fresh fruit
Sweet pickle	use less substitute a salad item, eg. tomato
Individual fruit pie	substitute fresh fruit
Chocolate	eat less substitute fresh fruit substitute low-sugar biscuit
Tomato ketchup	use less
Canned fruit	use fruit canned in natural juice substitute fresh fruit substitute fruit stewed in little or no sugar
Rice pudding	make it at home so the amount of sugar can be regulated substitute sugar reduced yoghurt
Coke	substitute fresh orange juice try sugar-reduced variety (low calorie Coke)

Checklist: 'Going Shopping'

The following table offers alternatives for high sugar foods:

Food with a high sugar content	Alternatives with a lower sugar content
Squashes, pop, fizzy drinks	Fresh fruit juice or those with reduced sugar content (low calorie version), water.
Sugar-coated breakfast cereals	Varieties without added sugar.
Muesli	Varieties without added sugar or try making your own.
Biscuits and cakes	Less sweet varieties Low sugar muesli bars Try making with less sugar than recipe states (many recipes are successful using half the sugar stated or using dried fruit for natural sweetness).
Fruit canned in sugar syrup	Fruit canned in natural juice.
Puddings	Fruit canned in natural juice Fresh fruit Sugar-reduced yoghurt Try making own rice pudding, custard, etc. using less sugar than usual.
Fruit yoghurt	Natural yoghurt and add fresh or stewed fruit to flavour. Sugar-reduced yoghurt. Fruit and natural yoghurts mixed. Natural yoghurt.
Ice cream	Yoghurt—try one of the suggestions above.
Jam, marmalade, etc.	Sugar-reduced varieties.
Sweets and chocolate	Fresh fruit Nuts Dried fruit
Foods with a high sugar content	Buy smaller quantities, less frequently.
Preserves, eg. pickles, chutneys	Sugar-reduced varieties, pickled vegetables.

Background Information: The Salt Picture

The chemical name for salt is sodium chloride. It is the sodium in this chemical which gives rise for concern when discussing salt in relation to health. It is, therefore, necessary to consider other sources of sodium in the diet, eg. bicarbonate of soda.

Sodium is found in food in a variety of forms. Some of the most common are salt, brine, baking powder, sodium bicarbonate, monosodium glutamate, sodium sulphite and other chemicals with the chemical symbol Na or compounds which contain sodium. It is as well to be aware, especially when reading food labels, of the variety of ways in which sodium can occur in the diet.

Some sodium is essential: in order for the body to function properly the correct balance between sodium and other body salts must be maintained. More sodium is needed under certain conditions such as heavy manual work or in very high temperatures. On average a person consumes about 12 grams of salt per day, ie. 2½ teaspoons. Under normal circumstances a person can remain healthy on much less salt, about ½ gram/day.

With most people excess sodium is excreted and there are no harmful effects. For some, excess sodium may cause high blood pressure, which means there is a risk of heart disease and strokes. As there is difficulty in determining those at risk, all individuals can be encouraged to reduce their intake of sodium. As salt is normally consumed to excess, this recommendation will not cause any harm and may be of benefit. The NACNE report recommends that salt intakes should fall on average by 3 grams per day.

Much of the sodium consumed comes from salt used in processing and preserving food, as well as that which is added by individuals.

Ways of reducing salt in the diet are as follows:

(a)   gradually cut down the amount added until none is added at all;
(b)   taste food before adding salt—it may not need any more;
(c)   use less salt in cooking—again, do this gradually;
(d)   be aware of foods which are high in salt (and/or sodium) and look at ways of reducing the quantity of such foods.

Salt substitutes can be used, eg. Selora, Lo-Salt. These substitutes are often made with potassium chloride. It is better to adjust one's taste to using less salt. Anyone with a heart or kidney condition should consult his general practitioner before using salt substitutes.

Sea salt, iodised salt, garlic salt and onion salt are still basically types of salt and cannot be used as substitutes.

Activity 3.6 will help individuals to become more aware of the foods which are high or low in salt and the reasons why this should be so.

Task Sheet: The Salt Picture

To leaders: Photocopy this sheet—cut out tasks one to four so they can be handed
separately to four small groups.

Task One

List (a) the types of food one would normally add salt to after preparation.
    (b) the types of food one would add salt to when cooking.
    (c) the types of food one would never add salt to.

Give the reasons for your answers.

Task Two

What kinds of food are to be found in the following food groups: meat, fruit, dairy
products and preserves?

Which of these foods might be high in salt and why?

Task Three

What kinds of food are to be found in the following food groups: fish, vegetables and
cereal foods?

Which of these foods might be high in salt and why?

Task Four

Suggest ways of making food to which no salt has been added (or contains no salty
ingredient, eg. yeast or beef extract) interesting and tasty.

Checklist: The Salt Picture

Task One

(a)   The types of food one would normally add salt to after preparation include eggs, meat, fish, chips, vegetables, salads and sandwich fillings.
Many people add salt to food without tasting it. Sometimes it is simply a matter of habit or custom. Some shake the salt cellar a consistent number of times regardless of how much salt comes out!

(b)   The types of food to which one would normally add salt when cooking include dishes with meat, fish, poultry, eggs, cheese, vegetables, pasta, rice, etc. In fact, most savoury dishes (and some cakes) have some salt added to them.

(c)   Salt is never (or very rarely) added to such foods as tinned fruit, fruit drinks, fruit yoghurt, tea, coffee or milk.

Tasks Two and Three

All the foods in the food groups will not contribute large amounts of sodium to the diet if eaten fresh. The salt content will increase if the foods are processed, preserved in salt, or if salt is added during cooking. Examples of foods which are high in salt are:

bacon	smoked haddock
ham	sardines
tongue	shell fish
corned beef	bottled sauces
luncheon meat	pickles
sausages	chutneys
kippers	

cheese, especially Danish blue, Stilton and processed cheese
vegetables canned in salt, food preserved in brine
commercially-produced cakes and biscuits
some breakfast cereals
snacks, eg. crisps and other nibbles
yeast and beef extracts

Task Four

Taste buds soon adjust to less salt in foods. In fact, if less salt is used the true flavour of the food can be enjoyed. The use of herbs, spices, peppers, a variety of dressings, eating vegetables raw, cooking vegetables for the shortest possible time and adding lemon juice in place of salt are all ways of making food interesting and tasty.

SESSION FOUR

Session Four

Contents   Session Plan

Group Material:
    Task Sheet: Mix and Match
    Task Sheet: Dietary Fibre in Your Food
Leader's Material:
    Background Information: Dietary Fibre
    Instructions: Mix and Match
    Checklist: Mix and Match
    Checklist: Dietary Fibre in Your Food
    Suggestions for Dietary Fibre Quiz: How Many Do You Know?

Aids   Flip-chart/OHP/Ts
Felt-tip pens, pens, pencils
Selection of foods containing fibre for quiz
Writing paper

Objectives 1 To understand the meaning of the term 'dietary fibre'.
        2 To understand the possible role for fibre in preventing some health problems.
        3 To know which foods are good sources of fibre.
        4 To be aware of less familiar sources of fibre, eg. pulses.

Many people think that they know what is meant by the term 'dietary fibre'. In reality, some misconceptions still occur: the term 'fibre' is sometimes confused with muscle fibre. The introductory explanation of the meaning of 'dietary fibre' in Activity 4.1 by the group leader will ensure that any misconceptions are clarified at the beginning of the session.

The task 'Mix and Match' enables the group to explore the possibility that fibre in the diet can help to prevent the occurrence of some health problems. As this exercise will generate much interesting discussion about the problems used as examples and as it is likely that a variety of other issues relating to fibre may be raised, it may be helpful for group leaders to read up on fibre before the session.

The 'Fibre in Your Food' chart (Activity 4.3) is intended to provide the group with some ideas about good and poor sources of fibre. When the exercise has been completed the chart may be taken home and used for reference.

The final activity (Activity 4.4) 'How many do you know' reinforces the previous one. A selection of foods containing fibre are displayed; some of these will be unfamiliar to group members. Possible items for inclusion are given in the group leader's information for the fibre quiz.

SESSION PLAN

Activity number	Activity/time	Organisation, methods and content
4.1	DIETARY FIBRE WHAT IT IS AND WHAT IT DOES 10 minutes	(a) Leader asks group what they understand by the term 'dietary fibre'. Leader clarifies any misconceptions and explains term fully. (b) Leader explains the various functions of fibre (see background information). It may be helpful to have the functions written on a flip-chart and displayed throughout the session.
4.2	MIX AND MATCH A HEALTHY ROLE FOR FIBRE 40 minutes	(a) Group members work in pairs. Leader distributes 'Mix and Match' task sheets—one to each pair. (b) Leader explains how to carry out the exercise (see instructions on task sheets). Group members complete the task. (c) Full group re-forms. Leader checks answers and discusses points raised with full group.
4.3	DIETARY FIBRE IN YOUR FOOD 20 minutes	(a) Group members work individually. Each member is handed a chart 'Fibre in Your Food' to complete. (b) When charts have been completed leader asks group members in turn for their responses to each food. (c) Leader comments appropriately. Group discusses findings from exercise.

Activity number	Activity/time	Organisation, methods and content
4.4	QUIZ—HOW MANY DO YOU KNOW? 20 minutes	(a) Group works in pairs. (b) Leader indicates display and asks pairs to see how many items they recognise. (c) Group re-forms. Leader discloses correct identity of each food. (d) Discuss in full group, as time permits.

Background Information: Dietary Fibre

Dietary fibre (or roughage as it used to be called) is a term used to describe a complex group of carbohydrates found mainly in the cell walls of plants. These substances act as a skeleton which supports the plant by giving it strength and shape. Dietary fibre is present in foods of vegetable origin only.

Many foods now undergo much processing which may remove fibre as well as vitamins and minerals. One of the best examples of this is the use of refined flour in making bread, biscuits and cakes. The consumption of refined foods has greatly contributed to the depletion of fibre in the diet and possibly to the increase of some of the 'western' health problems of today.

The NACNE Report recommends that the intake of fibre in the average British diet should be increased from 20 grams per day to 30 grams. Where changes are desirable, these should be gradual to allow the body to adjust to this new way of eating. Another adjustment which may have to be made is an increase in the amount of fluid taken. At least 1–1½ litres of fluid needs to be consumed daily. (Fluid can be taken as water, fruit juice, beverages, etc.). This is because high-fibre foods absorb fluid as they pass through the digestive system.

The best way to increase the intake of fibre is to eat more of the foods which are naturally high in fibre. Examples of such foods are wholemeal bread, wholegrain cereals, vegetables and fruit. It is preferable to increase the fibre intake by eating more of these foods than by adding large quantities of bran to a refined diet. Bran is the husk of the cereal grain and provides fibre in a highly concentrated form.

Although fibre passes through the digestive system largely undigested it performs a variety of essential functions which may help to prevent the occurrence of some health problems. Some of the main functions of fibre are as follows:

1   Fibre increases the bulk and softness of the stools because it absorbs fluid as it passes through the digestive system.
2   The increased bulk stimulates the action of the bowel (peristalsis), thus making the stools easier to pass.
3   Fibre reduces the length of time food takes to pass through the digestive system; this is known as the transit time.
4   Food which contains fibre requires more chewing and has a higher degree of satiety.
5   Fibre slows down the absorption of carbohydrate. Consequently, there is a much more gradual increase of blood sugar levels after the intake of food which is high in fibre. In cases where the diet is highly refined, the absorption of sugar is much more rapid.

The Preventive Role of Fibre

1   *Constipation*: A diet which has a high-fibre content can help to treat and prevent constipation. Dietary fibre, especially that obtained from cereal sources, decreases the transit time and increases the bulk and softness of the stools.

2   *Haemorrhoids*: A high-fibre diet leads to softer stools and therefore less straining when opening the bowels: this can reduce the symptoms of haemorrhoids.

3   *Diverticular disease*: Diverticula are small pouches in the wall of the large bowel (colon). They may arise as a result of a low-fibre diet causing increased pressure on the colon wall, thus forcing out the wall to form small pockets. These small pockets are called diverticula and it is in these where some bowel contents may collect. Diverticulitis is the inflammation of the diverticula which can cause pain and diarrhoea. A high-fibre diet can help to relieve the symptoms of diverticular disease and may help to prevent it.

4   *Cancer of the large bowel*: A high fibre diet may be a protective factor against cancer of the large bowel by:
     (a)   increasing the bulk of the stools, thus diluting the concentration of possible carcinogens;
     (b)   reducing the transit time of the food passing through the intestines. This reduces the exposure time to possible carcinogens.

5   *Diabetes mellitus*: Fibre helps to slow down the absorption of sugar from the small bowel. This, in turn, helps to prevent wide and rapid fluctuations of blood sugar levels and so aids the regulation of the condition.

6   *Obesity*: Foods which are high in fibre may help to prevent and treat obesity by being more satisfying and requiring more chewing than refined foods. People tend to eat less of bulkier high-fibre foods as they become 'full up' more quickly than when eating refined foods. Those who eat highly refined foods may soon feel hungry again as their blood sugar level rises rapidly and then falls quickly. It is thus likely that they will consume more food.

Task Sheet: Mix and Match

Column 1	Column 2	Column 3	Column 4
Health problem	Matching letters and numbers	Description of health problem	Possible role of fibre in prevention
Constipation		1 Swollen veins in the walls of anus.	(a) Foods which contain fibre require more chewing and are more satisfying.
Diverticular disease		2 A condition caused by the non-production or under-production of insulin by the pancreas.	(b) Fibre absorbs water as it passes through the intestines which increases the bulk and softness of the stools.
Haemorrhoids		3 A health problem which occurs when a person is 20% over the desirable weight for their height.	(c) Fibre reduces the length of time it takes for the food to pass through the digestive system.
Cancer of the large bowel		4 There is difficulty in passing stools: infrequent hard small stools are produced.	(d) Fibre slows down the absorption of sugar. There is a much slower increase of levels of blood sugar after a high-fibre meal.
Diabetes mellitus		5 The presence of small pouches in the wall of the large bowel.	(e) The increased bulk stimulates the action of the bowel (peristalsis) thus making the stools easier to pass.
Obesity		6 The presence of a malignant tumour in the large bowel.	

Instructions: 'Mix and Match'

How to Mix and Match

The task is to match the health problem from Column One to its description from Column Three and the possible role which fibre may play in prevention from Column Four. When the appropriate columns are matched the answers are put in the boxes in Column Two.

There is only *one* description for each health problem stated in Column Three *but* there may be *more than one role* from Column Four which applies to a single health problem.

Example: If you think that the correct description for constipation is Item One from Column Three and roles (a) and (c) from Column Four then the answers would go in the boxes in Column Two as follows:

1	a	c	

The matching process is complete when the descriptions and the possible preventive roles of fibre have been correctly matched to all six health problems.

Checklist: 'Mix and Match'

Column 1 Health problem	Column 2 Matching letters and numbers
Constipation	4 b c e
Diverticular disease	5 b c e
Haemorrhoids	1 b e
Cancer of the large bowel	6 b c
Diabetes mellitus	2 d
Obesity	3 a d

Task Sheet: Dietary Fibre in Your Food

Listed below are some everyday foods. Tick the column that you feel indicates the appropriate fibre value of that food, if an average-sized portion is consumed.

Food	Good source of fibre	Poor source of fibre	No fibre content
Banana			
Tomatoes			
Bran cereal			
White bread/chapati			
Milk			
Apple			
Wheat biscuit cereal			
Meat			
Brown rice			
Cucumber			
Baked potatoes			
Lentils/dhal			
Cornflakes			
Wholewheat pasta			
Brown bread/chapati			
Eggs			
Peas, processed			
Boiled potatoes			
Orange			
Rye crispbread			
Wholemeal bread/chapati			
Carrots			
Spring greens			
Dried fruit eg. sultanas			
White rice			
Beans, baked			
Peanuts			
Cream crackers			
Sugar			
Grapes			
Fish			
Yam			

Checklist: Dietary Fibre in Your Food

For the purpose of this exercise the foods have been placed in the categories indicated according to the following criteria:

Good source of fibre—more than 2.0g fibre per portion
Poor source of fibre—less than 2.0g fibre per portion
No fibre content.

Food	Portion size	Dietary fibre content per portion	Category
Banana	150g	3.0g	Good
Tomatoes	60g	0.9g	Poor
Bran cereal	50g	13.3g	Good
White bread/chapati	60g	1.6/2.0g	Poor
Milk	1 glass	Nil	No fibre
Apple	120g	2.4g	Good
Wheat biscuit cereal	30g	3.8g	Good
Meat	80g	Nil	No fibre
Brown rice (raw weight)	60g	2.5g	Good
Cucumber	60g	0.2g	Poor
Baked potatoes (baked in skins)	150g	3.0g	Good
Lentils (dhal)	120g	4.4g	Good
Cornflakes	30g	0.9g	Poor
Wholewheat pasta (raw weight)	60g	6.0g	Good
Brown bread/chapati	60g	3.1g/4.0g	Good
Eggs	1	Nil	No fibre
Peas—processed	120g	9.5g	Good
Boiled potatoes	120g	1.2g	Poor
Orange	180g	2.7g	Good
Rye crispbread	30g	3.5g	Good
Wholemeal bread/chapati	60g	5.1g/6.1g	Good
Carrots	120g	3.6g	Good
Spring greens	90g	3.4g	Good
Dried fruit eg. sultanas	30g	2.1g	Good
White rice (raw weight)	60g	1.4g	Poor
Beans—baked	120g	8.8g	Good
Peanuts	30g	2.4g	Good
Cream crackers	30g	0.9g	Poor
Sugar	10g	Nil	No fibre
Grapes	120g	1.1g	Poor
Fish	120g	Nil	No fibre
Yam	90g	3.7g	Good

Suggestions for Dietary Fibre Quiz: How Many Do You Know?

The purpose of this quiz is to introduce the group members to fibre-containing foods. It is suggested that the display should not only include foods with which they are likely to be familiar, but also foods that are less commonplace but which are equally useful sources of fibre.

Some suggestions for foods which could be included in the fibre quiz are given below:

Wholemeal bread	Baked beans
Wholemeal chapatis	Oranges
Brown rice	Apples
Wholemeal pasta	Carrots
Red kidney beans	Muesli
Mung beans	Wheat biscuit cereal
Soya beans	Lentils—a variety
Wholemeal flour	Rye crispbread
Dried fruit	Butter beans
Nuts	Puffed wheat
Black-eyed beans	

Reminder

Fruit and vegetables provide a useful source of vitamins and minerals as well as dietary fibre especially when eaten raw. Some fruit and vegetables should be included in the display to emphasise their role in healthy eating.

SESSION FIVE

Session Five

Contents   Session Plan

Group Material:
  Fatty Dip—Master Copy
Leader's Material:
  Checklist: Fat—Where Are You?
  Background Information: Fat—Who Needs It?

Group Project:
  Making and Tasting Healthy Dishes.

Aids   Flip-chart/OHP/Ts
Container for 'Fatty Dip'
Pens/pencils
Writing paper
Paper for display of 'A Day's Healthy Eating'

Objectives   1   To identify foods which are high in fat.
2   To know the reasons for including some fat in the diet.
3   To know the health problems associated with high-fat diets.
4   To identify alternatives to high-fat foods.
5   To plan a day of healthy eating.
6   To enable group members to clarify important points about healthy eating.
7   To discuss ideas for a group project with group members.

This session focuses on the role of fat in the diet. The first exercise (Activity 5.1) 'Fat—Where Are You?' is used as both a warm-up for the session and to enable the group to become aware of the wide variety of foods which contain fat.

It seems to be a fairly common misconception that "if fat is 'bad for you' wouldn't it be better to cut it out all together?". It is important that group members should understand the need to include some fat in their daily eating—whilst at the same time realising the health risks associated with too much fat. 'Fat—Who Needs It?' (Activity 5.2) provides an opportunity for members to discuss these points.

In order to look at ways of reducing fat in the diet an exercise called 'Fatty Dip' (Activity 5.3) has been devised. A master sheet is provided which can be photocopied to provide examples of high-fat foods. This activity usually generates interest in ways of reducing fat intake and the ideas produced can then be discussed.

In order to relate this next exercise (Activity 5.4) to everyday life, the group works in pairs to devise a day of healthy eating which is relevant to one or both members of the pair. It is likely that in any group there will be a wide variety of eating patterns which are influenced by culture, income, age, life style, etc. The day's intake can be for a family, someone living on his own, someone at school all day. The possibilities are endless—the principles are still the same. Group members will need to bear in mind the information about sugar, salt and fibre that they have acquired in the previous sessions, as well as the points raised about fat in this one.

Hints and tips (Activity 5.5) is linked with the material in Activity 5.4. It provides an opportunity for group members to assess what they consider to be the most important aspects of healthy eating.

The final activity in this session is the preparation of the Group Project (Activity 5.6). A full explanation of how this may be carried out is found in the text on page 85.

SESSION PLAN

Activity number	Activity/time	Organisation, methods and content
5.1	FAT—WHERE ARE YOU? 10 minutes	(a) *Brainstorm* to produce a list of foods which contain fat. (b) Leader asks group 'What have you learned from this exercise?'
5.2	FAT—WHO NEEDS IT? 15 minutes	(a) Leader explains why fat is needed in the diet. (b) Group works in small groups. (c) Leader explains that too much fat in the diet may lead to health problems. (d) Leader asks group to list possible health problems associated with too much fat. (e) Group re-forms. Leader receives feedback and discusses appropriately.
5.3	FATTY DIP 10 minutes	(a) Leader explains exercise (see notes on top of master copy). (b) Group completes round of alternatives to high-fat food. Leader to comment as necessary.

78

Activity number	Activity/time	Organisation, methods and content
5.4	HEALTHY EATING 25 minutes	(a) Group works in pairs. (b) Leader asks pairs to plan a day of healthy eating which is relevant to one or both members of each pair. The plans should take into account the previous exercises on reducing fat in this session *and* the nutritional recommendations on sugar, salt and fibre covered in previous sessions. (c) Pairs to display plans on flip-chart paper/large sheets of paper around the room. (d) Leader and group members to comment and to discuss plans when displayed.
5.5	HINTS AND TIPS 20 minutes	(a) Group works in small groups. (b) Leader asks groups to list five of the most important hints and tips they would like to give to a friend who is interested in healthy eating. (Allow about 10 minutes for this task.) (c) Small groups to report back to full group. Discuss briefly, as time allows.
5.6	PREPARATION FOR GROUP PROJECT 10 minutes	(a) Leader explains project to group and allows group to discuss how project will be carried out. Final arrangements to be made in next session.

Checklist: Fat—Where Are You?

It is unlikely that the group will have any difficulty in naming foods which are high in fat. It may be more difficult for them to identify foods which contain 'hidden' fat. The purpose of this exercise is to encourage the group to identify these foods as in the similar exercise 'Hidden sugar in foods' in Session Three.

The following may be given as examples of high-fat foods:

Biscuits (including cracker types)
Scones
Cakes
Pastries
Chocolate
Some puddings, eg. cake and pastry mixtures, cheesecake
Ice-cream
Cheese dishes
Egg dishes
Chapatis made with fat
Vegetable oils
Meats
Sausages
Meat products, eg. luncheon meat
Crisps
Chips
French dressing
Mayonnaise
Salad cream.

Background Information: Fat—Who Needs It?

The NACNE Report recommends that the fat intake should be, on average, 30% of total energy intake. Fat currently supplies approximately 40% of total energy in the average British diet. The recommendation is, therefore, a reduction not an exclusion of fat. Health problems can result if the diet is too high in fat or if it lacks it completely.

The NACNE Report also recommends that the saturated fatty acid intake should be reduced from 18% of the total energy intake to 10%. Saturated fatty acids are mainly derived from animal fats and some vegetable fats (eg. coconut and palm oil). By encouraging group members to reduce total fat, especially from dairy fat and meat fat, the saturated fatty acid intake will be reduced at the same time as a total fat reduction. This aspect of fat reduction may be developed throughout the session depending upon the needs of the group.

Reasons for Including Fat in the Diet

1   Fat provides a valuable source of fat-soluble vitamins, A, D, E and K.
2   Fats are necessary to provide the essential polyunsaturated fatty acids needed by the body. Only a few grams of these essential fatty acids are required per day: most people eat far in excess of this amount.
3   Fat has a high energy value, approximately twice that of protein or carbohydrate. Its presence in the diet will reduce the bulk of food needed to make up the total dietary energy. This is an advantage to very young children and to those whose life style necessitates a high energy intake. For others, the concentrated energy in high-fat foods may lead to taking in more energy than the body needs and so to excess weight.
4   The body store of fat is used for energy and warmth when required. Fat stored under the skin helps to regulate the body temperature.
5   Fat is used to protect the vital organs, eg. the heart and the kidneys.

Reasons for Reducing Fat in the Diet

1   A high-fat diet, particularly one which is high in saturated fat, is associated with ischaemic heart disease (IHD). Many experts believe that a major contributor of IHD is a high level of blood cholesterol. A diet which is high in fat may lead to high blood levels of cholesterol and to atherosclerosis. Both factors have an effect on the risk of IHD.
2   The high energy value of fat often means that a high-fat diet may lead to a person becoming overweight. This, in turn, increases the risk of associated problems such as heart disease, gallbladder problems, diabetes mellitus, respiratory problems and skin infections.

Note: It is important that skimmed milk should not be given to children under the age of five years. There can be a progressive introduction of semi-skimmed milk after the age of two years **providing that the child's overall dietary intake is adequate**.

Fatty Dip—Master Copy

To the Leader:

Photocopy this sheet, cut the large square into individual rectangular slips, each one bearing the name of a high-fat food, fold the slips and put them into a container. You are now ready to play Fatty Dip.

Pass the container round group until all slips have been taken. Ask full group to complete a round(s) of ''My high-fat food is . . . An alternative would be . . .''.

FULL-CREAM MILK	BUTTER	MARGARINE	CHOCOLATE
CHIPS	CHEESE	CUSTARD	FISH IN BATTER
DUMPLINGS	SALAD DRESSING	CREAM	BEEFBURGERS
FRIED FOOD	DOUGHNUTS	CRISPS	SAUSAGES
STEAMED SUET FRUIT PUDDING	MEAT	ROAST POTATOES	SAUCES

Checklist: 'Fatty Dip'

The following table lists high-fat foods for use in 'Fatty Dip' together with lower-fat alternatives:

High-fat foods for Fatty Dip	Lower-fat alternatives
Full-cream milk	Skimmed or semi-skimmed milk
Butter	Low-fat spreads, or use sparingly
Margarine	Low-fat spreads, or use sparingly
Cheese	Cottage cheese or lower-fat cheeses such as Edam, Gouda, Brie, Camembert. Try a strong flavoured cheese and use less
Cream	Low-fat yoghurt, ice cream or custard (make with skimmed milk), lower-fat cream alternative
Custard	Make with skimmed or semi-skimmed milk
Sauces	Use recipes which do not require added fat Make with skimmed milk or semi-skimmed milk or low-fat yoghurt For cheese sauce use lower-fat-content cheeses
Chocolate	Eat less or substitute fresh fruit
Salad dressing	Use recipes with low-fat yoghurt or try salads which do not need an oil or fatty dressing
Dumplings	More potato or dried beans or peas in casseroles/stews
Doughnut	Fresh/dried fruit
Steamed suet fruit pudding	Baked apple, stewed fruit, fruit crumble or fresh fruit
Crisps	Crackers and cottage cheese. Fresh or dried fruit
Fish in batter	Grilled, baked or poached fish Use oatmeal to coat, not batter

High-fat foods for Fatty Dip	Lower-fat alternatives
Meat	Grill Use less—drain fat off gravy Choose lean meat Use smaller quantities in casseroles/stews and add dried beans, peas or lentils Cut fat off before eating Eat poultry and fish more often and red meat less often Use more vegetable-based dishes
Sausages	Grill Try low-fat varieties Eat less frequently
Beefburgers	Grill Home-made beefburgers using lean meat
Chips	Jacket potato Boiled potato Brown rice Wholemeal pasta
Fried foods	Use another method of cooking such as grilling, baking, etc.
Roast potatoes	Use plain boiled or baked (jacket) potatoes Use alternatives such as rice and pasta depending on other foods served

Group Project: Making and Tasting Healthy Dishes

The main purpose of this exercise is to relate the principles of the course to food preparation. Leaders and group members should be looking for dishes which show either a decrease in the amount of sugar, salt and fat and/or an increase in the amount of fibre when compared with more traditional recipes.

There are various ways of carrying out the group project—some suggestions are given below. The method chosen will depend on how much the group wishes to contribute to the project (both financially and individually), the cooking facilities and other practical difficulties which may arise when introducing an activity of this nature. The methods presented here are those which have been found to work elsewhere.

Suggestions for Carrying Out Group Project

1   Group members select the dishes they would like to be prepared. Either a cookery demonstrator or one or more members of the group prepare and cook dishes in a group project session.

2   Each group member selects and prepares a dish which can be brought to the group project session. Group members should be encouraged to taste each other's dishes.

3   The group selects suitable dishes and one volunteer to prepare the dishes and bring them along to the group project session. All group members may taste the dishes.

4   Each group member brings a recipe for an inexpensive healthy dish. Recipe ideas to be exchanged.

The financing of this part of the course can be met in one of several ways:

(a)   Group members can make a small contribution at each session or one contribution to cover the cost of the project.

(b)   The cost of the dishes may be met by group funds (if applicable).

(c)   If the group belongs to an organisation, eg. church, parent/teacher association, the cost may be met from their funds.

(d)   If the group is associated with a voluntary organisation a small grant may be available.

(e)   Each group member could finance the cost of his selected dish.

SESSION SIX

Session Six

Contents   Session Plan

Group Material:
    Food Presentation—Master Copy
    Height/Weight Charts
Leader's Material:
    Background Information: 'On the Line'
    Checklist: Food Presentation

Aids   Flip-chart/OHP/Ts
Felt-tip pens
Envelopes containing food and drink appraisals from Session Two

Objectives 1 To examine the concept of healthy weight.
        2 To identify other factors which affect an individual's concept of weight.
        3 To re-examine the food and drink appraisals completed at the beginning of the course.
        4 To finalise the group project arrangements.
        5 To identify ways of presenting food attractively.

'On the Line' (Activity 6.1) is an exercise designed to enable group members to examine the concept of a healthy weight and to discuss the factors that may influence their perceptions of it.

As this is the penultimate session, it is an appropriate time for group members to re-examine the food and drink appraisal completed in Session Two. This activity (6.2) offers the opportunity for individuals to identify any changes they have made in their daily eating patterns and to assess what they have learned during the course.

The group project arrangements (Activity 6.3) are finalised during this session.

The food presentation exercise (Activity 6.4) forms the basis of a brief discussion in the value of presenting food attractively.

Activity number	Activity/time	Organisation, methods and content
6.1	ON THE LINE 35 minutes	(a) Leader explains exercise—see 'On the Line' leader's instructions. (b) Group carries out activity. (c) Group re-forms for discussion (see leader's instructions). (d) At an appropriate time, leader hands out height/weight charts to allow group to identify the range their own weight is in. (e) Leader asks group 'What have you learned from doing this exercise?'
6.2	LOOKING BACK 15 minutes	(a) Leader returns the appropriate envelope containing the food and drink appraisal completed in Session Two to each group member. (b) Group members review the content of their appraisal for a few minutes. (c) *Round*: ''One thing I have learned from reading my appraisal . . .'' (d) Full group discussion; leader comments appropriately.

Activity number	Activity/time	Organisation, methods and content
6.3	FINALISING GROUP PROJECT ARRANGEMENTS 30 minutes	(a) Leader discusses project with group in order to finalise arrangements for the following session. (b) Leader asks members if they would like to bring cookery books, recipes, or anything else of interest to the final session.
6.4	FOOD PRESENTATION 10 minutes	(a) Leader hands out one or more suggestions to group members for presenting food attractively. (b) *Round*: 'One way I could use this suggestion(s) is . . .' (c) Leader asks group if they think there is any value in presenting food attractively. (d) Full group discusses points raised as time permits.

HEIGHT/WEIGHT CHART

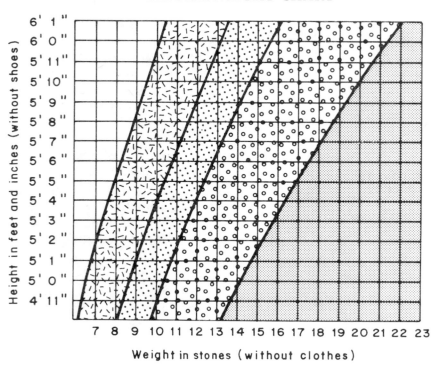

Key

☐ You are underweight and could do with a few extra pounds

▨ This is the ideal weight for your height

▦ You are getting fat so choose your food more carefully

▧ This is the danger sign. You are very overweight and need to lose weight. Your health could be suffering as a result.

▓ You are severely overweight and your health is in danger. It would be advisable to consult your doctor about your weight.

Take a line up from your weight and a line across from your height. The point of intersection will fall within your weight range. You will be able to tell which range you are in by reading the key.

Background Information: 'On the Line'

'On the Line' is an exercise based on the continuum activity outlined in the notes on participatory learning on page 8. In this case, the two extremes are 'Person A is very overweight' and 'Person B is very underweight'. In this session the term 'obese' has deliberately not been used as it is little understood by the general public. 'Very overweight' has been used in preference as it is a term which most people can easily relate to. Similarly, the 'underweight' end of the line has not been labelled (and should not be) 'Person B has anorexia nervosa'. Anorexia nervosa is a psychiatric disorder: a person who is underweight need not necessarily be anorexic.

This is a most interesting exercise which needs to be handled with some sensitivity and for this reason has been left until the group members know each other well. The activity produces much material for discussion. There are many surprises when group members learn how others perceive their own weight.

If leaders are at all apprehensive about using the exercise with their groups there are two alternatives:

(a)   the continuum line is drawn on a flip-chart or OHT and the group members can then write their names on it, or use different symbols if they wish;

(b)   the group members write their names on a piece of paper and place these on the imaginary line on the floor instead of physically standing there. It is thus the name on the paper which occupies the line position and it is the name which moves.

Discussion

How ever the activity is conducted, there is much to discuss when the full group re-forms. The points most likely to be raised by the group and/or the leader are:

(a)   the part of the line which represents a healthy weight range;
(b)   the role which self-image and appearance play in perceptions of a healthy weight;
(c)   the realisation that a healthy weight covers a range of weights and not one specific weight.

All of the discussion points will be reinforced and developed during the discussion. This activity will bring out factors which affect personal perceptions of weight such as advertising, exercise, weight loss, expectations of others, how I see myself, roles, age, job, etc.

Discussion can proceed as time allows. This exercise is a good foundation for ideas for future work if the group is to continue meeting.

The height/weight chart will clarify which range the group members are in as regards their weight. It may be useful to know of any activities which are available locally which may help individuals to change their weight if this is desirable.

Food Presentation—Master Copy

To the Leader:

The following garnishes can be used in a variety of ways to enhance the appearance of a dish or meal. Cut out each section, fold into two and place in a suitable container in order to carry out the activity in the same way as for Fatty Dip.

LEMON OR ORANGE	PARSLEY
OATS OR OATMEAL	TOMATO
CUCUMBER	LETTUCE
NUTS	FRUIT
DRIED FRUIT	YOGHURT
MINT	POTATO
RADISH	CARROT
GREEN PEPPER	WATERCRESS
MUSTARD AND CRESS	CHIVES
HERBS OR SPICES	BREAD OR BREADCRUMBS

Checklist: Food Presentation

The presentation of a meal or a dish can make quite a difference to how appealing and interesting it appears to be. An appetising aroma, varieties of flavour, colour and taste all help to make an interesting meal and to stimulate the digestive juices.

The following suggested garnishes can be used in a variety of ways to enhance the appearance of a dish or meal.

	Garnish	Suggestions for use
1	Lemon or orange	slices, finely shredded peel, grated peel, different shapes.
2	Parsley	chopped, used in sprigs, provides colour contrast.
3	Oats or oatmeal	can be toasted, provides texture and colour contrast.
4	Tomato	slices, halves, quarters, 'flowers', colour contrast.
5	Cucumber	slices, shapes, chunks, colour contrast.
6	Lettuce	whole leaves, shredded, colour contrast.
7	Nuts	toasted or roasted, texture and colour contrast.
8	Fruit	slices, shapes, colour contrast.
9	Dried fruit	colour, texture.
10	Yoghurt	colour contrast.
11	Mint	chopped, sprigs, colour contrast.
12	Potato	piped, browned, borders, shapes.
13	Radish	shapes, colour contrast.
14	Carrots	grated strips, chopped, sliced, shapes, colour contrast.
15	Watercress	sprigs, bunched, colour contrast.
16	Green peppers	chopped, sliced in rings, shredded, colour contrast.
17	Mustard and cress	colour contrast.
18	Chives	chopped, colour contrast.
19	Herbs or spices	colour contrast.
20	Bread or breadcrumbs	toasted topping, texture contrast.

SESSION SEVEN

Session Seven

This session is very much the responsibility of the group members and the activities arranged for it will have been planned earlier in the course. Although the session is very informal, there are still specific objectives which apply at this stage in order to provide a complete overview of healthy eating.

Contents   Session Plan

Aids   Paper plates
Tasting spoons
Recipe books
Whatever else the group wishes to share with the other group
members.

Objectives   1   To promote discussion about healthy eating by being involved in the group project.
2   To enable group members to identify the key points they have learnt during the programme.
3   To provide an opportunity for an informal evaluation of the course.

The final session is interesting and enjoyable. It has a role in bringing the learning points covered in the programme together, and provides an opportunity for new approaches to healthy eating to be shared.

Background information has not been included as it is impossible to cover the range of activities which will be generated nationwide. The group leader will easily be able to pick up on points raised by their group members, thus making this activity a very individual one.

An exchange of recipes may be a good idea at this point. Group members can bring an assortment of recipe books, reference books or cuttings from magazines to share with other group members, as discussed in Sessions 5 and 6.

In Activity 7.2, 'Something New?', there will have been plenty of activity to promote group discussion. The leader may wish to record the learning points on a flip-chart or maintain the informality of the session by allowing the group to discuss freely what they have learned on the course.

'Regrets and Appreciates' (Activity 7.3) is a suitable way to end any course (see section on participatory learning). Other activities may be substituted if the group leader considers them to be appropriate.

SESSION PLAN

Activity number	Activity/time	Organisation, methods and content
7.1	GROUP PROJECT 60 minutes	Group members carry out project and share items of interest brought in by members.
7.2	SOMETHING NEW? 20 minutes	(a) As a full group discuss group project and identify key learning points. (b) Leader to ask group how useful they have found the course.
7.3	REGRETS AND APPRECIATES 10 minutes	As a full group: *Round*: One thing I have regretted about the course and one thing I have appreciated.

Although this is the last session, the course need not end here. If the group members wish to extend the course they can arrange visits to local shops, supermarkets and food manufacturers. Ways of passing on the lessons learned can be discussed. All group members will have a part to play in informal education in their roles as citizens, parents, siblings, professionals. Women have a particularly important role in this respect as it is more usual for women to act as the 'gate-keeper' in the house. This aspect of women's roles could lead to exploring other approaches to food and health. Similarly, the changing role of women and men in relation to food could be explored.

Should the group wish to disband it may be useful to share information about other activities in the area which would be relevant. The venues for weight gain/weight loss groups may be useful to know. Some of the group may like to join a Look After Yourself! course which adopts an holistic approach to health: exercise, relaxation and stress management, healthy eating and social drugs*. Some members may wish to attend cookery classes or start or join a completely different kind of health group.

In schools, young people may like to be involved in cooking a healthy meal for some of their friends and teachers. They can undertake simple surveys of opportunities for healthy eating in their school, college or local community. The lessons learned could link into other subjects in the school curriculum. Parents may also like to become involved and it may be possible to arrange some sessions for young people and their parents or to start a parents' healthy eating group.

The above are suggestions; the possibilities are endless in their variety and potential for education. The authors hope that the material in this programme will stimulate ideas for future activities aimed at a positive approach to good health and nutrition education.

---

*For information about 'Look After Yourself!' Courses contact the Look After Yourself Project Centre, Christchurch College, Canterbury, Kent CT1 1QU, your local health education unit, or your local library.

BIBLIOGRAPHY

Bibliography

The following books and reports have been used for reference in compiling *Food in Focus*:

Brandes D & Philips H (1979) *The Gamester's Handbook*. London: Hutchinson

British Dietetic Association (1987) *Children's Diet and Change*. A Report of the Child Health & Nutrition Working Party.

Burkitt D (1983) *Don't Forget Fibre in Your Diet*. London: Martin Dunitz

Committee on Medical Aspects of Food Policy (1984) *Diet and Cardiovascular Disease*. London: HMSO

Davidson S, Passmore R, Brock JF & Truswell AS (1979) *Human Nutrition and Dietetics*. Edinburgh: Churchill Livingstone

Evans M & Satow A (1983) *Working with Groups*. London: Health Education Council (accompanying video available.)

Hansen M with Marsden J (1984) *E for Additives, The Complete E Number Guide*. London: Butterworths

Health Education Council (1984) *The Scientific Basis of Dental Health Education—A Policy Document*. London: Health Education Council

DHSS (1982) *Eating for Health*. London: HMSO

Jukes DJ (1984) *Food Legislation in the UK*. London: Butterworths

Maryon Davis A (1984) *Diet 2000*. London: Granada

Ministry of Agriculture, Fisheries and Food (1984) (revised) *Look at the Label*. London: HMSO

National Advisory Council for Nutrition Education (1983) *A Discussion Paper on Proposals for Nutritional Guidelines for Health Education*. London: Health Education Council

The Nutrition Sub-committee of the Medical Advisory Committee, British Diabetic Association (1983) *Dietary Recommendations for Diabetics for the 1980s*. London: British Diabetic Association

Open University (1985) *Healthy Eating*. Milton Keynes: Open University Press

Paul AA & Southgate DAT (1979) *McCance & Widdowson's The Composition of Foods*. London: HMSO

Rice W (1981) *Informal Methods of Health and Social Education*. Manchester: TACADE

Royal College of Physicians (1980) *Medical Aspects of Dietary Fibre*. London: Pitman Medical

Wright M (1984) *The Salt Counter*. London: Pan Books